NEIL SPECTOR, M.D.

GONE IN A
HEARTBEAT

A Physician's Search for True Healing

For information contact Triton Press, 426 South Lamar Blvd., Suite 16, Oxford, MS 38655.

ISBN: 978-1-936-946-42-6

Triton Press
A division of The Nautilus Publishing Company
426 South Lamar Blvd., Suite 16
Oxford, Mississippi 38655
Tel: 662-513-0159
www.nautiluspublishing.com
www.neilspector.com

First Edition

Front cover design by Le'Herman Payton.
Front cover illustrations by Thinkstock Images

A special thanks to the Fluency Organization, Inc. in Tyler, Texas.

This book is not intended as a substitute for the medical advice of your physician. The reader should regularly consult a physician in matters relating to his/her health and particularly with respect to any symptoms that may require diagnosis or medical attention.

Printed in the United States of America

To my wife Denise, who I love and adore with all my heart and soul, and whose constant love and support is the reason I am alive today; to our daughter Celeste, who is the light and joy of our lives and a long awaited answer to our prayers; to my parents whose unconditional love shaped who I am today; to our families, our extended network of friends, neighbors, and prayer groups who never gave up hope and are a blessing to our lives; to Vicky and her family who will forever remain in my thoughts and prayers; and to those waiting for the gift of life: Have Faith!

To Eileen Barton for her thoughtful comments during the genesis of the book, and to Mary Ann Lackland (Fluency Organization) for her friendship and invaluable guidance and expertise in helping to realize my dream of publishing my story.

1

"Do you want me to sugarcoat this or just tell it like it is?" the head of transplant surgery said, standing at the foot of my bed.

I'd never met him before, but I had been around surgeons enough to know that they usually don't sweet talk. My wife, Denise, sat in the chair next to my bed.

"Tell me straight," I said.

"You'll be dead by Monday unless you have a heart transplant."

He paused while his words sunk in. There was one other option, he told us. They could implant a biventricular assist device in my abdomen to take the pressure off my failing heart. It would keep me alive, but I would not only be confined to my bed, but also connected to an external control unit the size of a small refrigerator.

"If you don't let us do something," he said, "you're not going to see Monday."

That was Friday afternoon on July 17, 2009. I was fifty-three years old. As the surgeon said those words, I felt a peaceful sensation. I should have been distraught over the prospect of my death, but for the first time in over 16 years I felt completely at ease. I put my head back on the pillow and smiled.

"Transfer me to Duke," I said.

Sometime in the next 72 hours I was going to have a heart transplant. Or I was going to die.

But my instincts told me that something miraculous was about to happen.

• • •

The heart palpitations had started 16 years earlier. I had never smoked, my family had no history of heart disease, I took my prophylactic baby aspirin once a day, and I drank a glass of red wine every now and then for the health benefits. My physical condition until the fall of 1993 had been superb. I ran 10-12 miles a day, six days a week, along the Charles River in Boston — something I had done religiously for years. I had even completed two Boston marathons — one in 1988 and the most recent in 1992.

Throughout the ensuing fall and winter of 1993, I began noticing frequent, transient episodes of a very rapid heart rate. Sometimes they lasted only a few seconds; others were longer.

Everyone has experienced a fast heart rate now and then. Perform strenuous exercise and your heart rate will accelerate from 70 beats per minute to 120 beats. It's a normal response. However, there was something strange about the episodes I was having. They might occur while I was relaxing, without any provocation. They were frightening enough that I drove myself to the emergency room several times, but by the time I was evaluated, my heart rate would have returned to normal.

With each evaluation came the usual reassurance that my heart was fine. Stress was most likely the culprit. After all, the doctors reminded me, I was a thirty-seven year old research physician under a great deal of pressure at work. In addition, my wife and I had recently moved from Boston to Florida, and we were trying to start a family.

Perhaps I should have felt relief at the doctors' explanations, but I did not. I instinctively knew that my condition was not stress-related. As an internal medicine resident, I had often worked 120-hour weeks in an extremely stressful environment and had never experienced anything like this. I was increasingly convinced that something else, a condition yet to be diagnosed, was responsible. But what was that "something"? Test after test failed to identify the cause of my symptoms, which only served to strengthen my doctors' resolve that stress had to be the culprit. The clock was ticking, and I felt certain that if I did not get an answer soon, the situation would get a lot worse.

I was, in fact, under pressure as so many Americans are today. I tried lowering my stress levels through different behavioral techniques, including meditation, biofeedback to control my heart rate and blood pressure, among other nontraditional techniques. But the heart palpitations persisted. They could happen anytime, anyplace—sitting still, driving, or taking a nap. I was at an impasse. My doctors were confident in their diagnosis.

My instincts told me they were wrong.

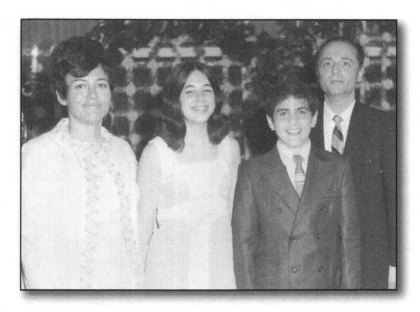

The Spector family

2

For the past 27 years, medicine has been a dominant part of my life: four years as a medical student, then three years as an internal medicine resident, followed by four years of specialized training in medical oncology, hematology, and bone marrow transplant. The remainder of my medical career I'd spent as an attending medical oncologist and hematologist.

Interestingly, being a physician had not been a lifelong ambition. Like many young boys, I had always dreamed of starring in the big leagues, hitting a home run in the bottom of the ninth inning with two outs and the score tied, to win the World Series. I wanted to be like Al Kaline, my childhood hero and star of the Detroit Tigers baseball team.

My parents were not the type who had planned my future. They simply wanted me to enjoy life and to be passionate about whatever career path I chose. My father was a rather brilliant scientist steeped in the traditions of the scientific method, where hypotheses were tested under controlled experimental conditions. My mother was an equally brilliant psychologist and family therapist — the consummate student of human behavior, which is often based on subjectivity rather than objectivity. The foundation was set. I owed my scientific inquisitiveness and my compassion to both my parents. They were the best role models anyone could have hoped for in life.

As a child, our family would go to the movies like other families. However, our movie nights were somewhat unusual. My father was a scientist at the National Institutes of Health in Bethesda, Maryland, the nation's research and clinic center. The auditorium on the top of the former NIH Clinical Center served as a movie theatre where patients, their families, and staff could watch free movies. My mother, sister, and I would watch movies while my dad would steal away to his lab to finish working, joining us after the film's credits.

Since NIH is a referral center for some of the most challenging cases in the world, my sister and I were guaranteed to see bizarre sights on our visits. My parents thought it important to expose us to children who were not as fortunate as we were. We often shared a play area with boys and girls suffering from rare diseases. It was not uncommon to play with kids our own age who were wearing football helmets because of neurological disorders so severe they might injure themselves.

The beauty of being exposed at such a young age to the NIH patients was that my sister and I never considered them any different from ourselves. I only took notice when a football helmet might have been from one of my favorites teams. I was never scared that the same fate of dying before my time might be in my future. I was simply fascinated by their diseases, and I remember questioning my father on why there wasn't more that could be done to help them.

On the other hand, many of our neighbors thought it was unhealthy that we were allowed to play with kids with such mysterious diseases. Where other children might be uncomfortable with physical deformities, gawking at them and making jokes as children are prone to do, my sister and I saw them as our playmates.

When I wasn't pretending to be Al Kaline, I loved standing beside my father in his lab watching him conduct experiments. Every once in a while, he allowed me my own research project. I was fascinated by the milieu of the laboratory. It was all so high-tech and important, although I didn't have a clue what he was actually doing. I just knew that his work was going to help people—a lot of people who were very sick.

My dad was a humble man, never one to brag about his accomplishments. I later discovered while taking a biochemistry course in medical school that his work at NIH was instrumental in discovering an enzyme in the body that controls the production of adrenaline and noradrenaline, hormones that help regulate blood vessel tone and cardiac function. His seminal findings led to the development of a new generation of drugs for the treatment of hypertension.

· · ·

Things came relatively easy for me in life. As a teenager, I performed well in sports and academics. When it came time for college, I attended my first choice: the University of North Carolina-Chapel Hill. Given that I was an out-of-state student, a rare commodity at UNC, I was grateful to be admitted. College brought plenty of sports and academics, along with some parties. And although they were four fun-filled and in some respects carefree years, I still managed to focus on my future.

I had entered college wanting to pursue one of three different career paths — medicine, clinical psychology, or the diplomatic core. But I chose medicine.

As a pre-med student, I majored in psychology and minored in zoology. During this time I volunteered at one of the state psychiatric hospitals, where I saw the devastation of chronic illness firsthand. Patients were incapacitated not by cancer or heart disease, but by voices in their heads. Like so many others with chronic medical conditions, they needed a tender touch and a sympathetic listener as much as they needed prescriptions.

That's when I knew medicine was the right choice for me. When confronted with serious illness (including psychiatric illness), a physician was likely to see people for who they really were. All of the false pretenses and bravado were wiped away. It left a rare opportunity to glimpse, authentically, into an individual's life. When patients understand that life is fragile — without guarantees from one day to the next — or when confronted with their own mortality, they tend to ask important, big questions about the meaning of life. And often about whether life after death exists.

I felt privileged that I might be someone patients could open up to and share their sorrow and laughter. Being a doctor would mean I could help people heal, not just physically, but emotionally. I was already beginning to realize that there is so much more to true healing than just taking medication.

Even those destined to die of their disease need to heal free of torment and live the remainder of their lives — whether measured in weeks, months, or years — in peace. That's what drove me into nearly three decades of medicine.

For me, it was the perfect choice. A choice that combined the traits passed along by both my parents.

Keeping those goals in mind during four years of medical school — years marked by long hours of studying, living off of junk food, and trying to retain my sanity in the midst of insanity — would prove to be quite different from my life up to this point.

Nothing about it would come easily.

3

It's been said that physicians only retain about five percent of what they are taught in medical school. I don't know if there is scientific merit underlying that figure, but it seemed reasonable to me, especially in light of my first two years of medical school. Each day brought more didactic lectures with an astronomical amount of information thrown at us.

The first two years, they say, prepare you for the last two years, which are nothing short of hell. In retrospect, those last two years were a haze, marked by chronic sleep deprivation and stress over never knowing quite enough to satisfy our attending physicians.

New Jersey Medical School was in the heart of downtown Newark, a city that still hadn't recovered from the 1967 race riots. The school itself was surrounded by tenements — many boarded up and harboring a clandestine world of gangs and crack addicts. Driving home late at night, I learned not to stop at red lights.

To make extra money, I spent nights working in the university hospital as part of the intravenous team. Students looking to make extra pocket change roamed the hospital from 6:00 pm to 6:00 am, checking on patients with intravenous lines (IVs), adjusting flow rates (these were the days prior to automatic IV infusion machines), and changing bags of fluids. We made rounds four times during the 12-hour shift, which usually meant covering at least 100 patients. There was little time — if any — for sleep. By the time I finished making rounds and starting new IVs, it was almost time to start rounds all over again. The few precious minutes of free time were spent studying for exams.

One of the benefits of being on the IV team was that it broke up the monotony of the first two years of coursework with some direct patient contact. I got to know patients and their families. In the midst of the insane schedule, it validated my career choice. I was often the one person on the team that patients and their families interacted with most often during the night. They asked questions about their disease. They discussed their fears. They cried on my shoulder. They were overcome with joy when things improved. I became a surrogate health care provider since they were often in the hospital for prolonged periods. It gave me a chance to see their disease progression or recovery.

I vividly remember one mother sitting vigil over her son, a young man in his mid-twenties. An aneurysm had ruptured in his brain, leaving him comatose. She stayed by his bedside every night for over a year, praying he would open his eyes just one more time. One night, I came in to check his IV, as I had done so many times before, but this time I witnessed a miracle. Her son was sitting up in bed, totally alert. His mother turned and embraced me as if I were a part of the family. In a strange way I felt it too.

My third and fourth years of medical school arrived just in time. It was becoming more difficult with every lecture to delay the gratification of being in the clinic with patients. Years three and four were especially difficult, both physically and emotionally. The time involved intense clinical rotations between internal medicine, surgery, psychiatry, and pediatrics services, with shorter rotations on emergency room medicine and some surgical subspecialties like orthopedics and ear/nose/throat. This broad range of experiences was designed to help us choose which area we wanted to pursue.

As third year students, we were the lowest on the hospital's totem pole. The residents often referred to us as "scut puppies." Get this! Do that! Clean this! Their demands were endless. It was a rite of passage, and I recall much of my medical training as something like being in the Marine Corps. We lived to please the residents who had just gone through the gauntlet themselves and were now taking their turn making us suffer.

There was very little time to stop and think about the patients as human beings. What they were thinking? What fears did they have? How had their illness affected their relationships with loved ones?

We were in survival mode: moving down the halls, studying, and getting a few precious hours of sleep whenever possible. Running, it seemed as if we were always running somewhere. I can remember often praying, Please God, just get me through the next two years.

For some reason I'd had this notion that someone would take the time to help us deal with the stress of being constantly surrounded by human misery, the stench of death clinging to our clothes. Every day for two years, we dealt with the anguish of patients grieving. Some were my own age when they were suddenly confronted by horrible, unexpected diseases.

Weren't there psychiatrists or psychologists who cared about the well-being of the medical students, I wondered? If so, where were they? Where was our help? I guess it wasn't considered important enough to be included in our training, although we were physically and emotionally drained and usually sleeping less than four hours a night, if that. We were never coached on how to communicate bad news to others. How would you tell a mother that her five-year-old is going to die? At least priests and rabbis have some training in this area. As medical students, we had none. Here, we learned by trial and error. God help anyone who receives life-altering bad news from inexperienced doctors-in-training who are merely trying to survive every day.

We were so unlike any other typical student fresh out of college. We did not have time to go to beer parties — okay, maybe a few — or football games on the weekends. Most of my other college friends were settling down by then. They had found good jobs, gotten married, and were buying homes. Meanwhile, I was routinely watching people cry over the death of a spouse, a parent, or a child. Who at twenty-five years is emotionally prepared to deal with this? It was raw emotion, human nature stripped to the bone without any pretenses. Death is death whether you are a multi-millionaire or you live on food stamps. It is gut wrenching. There are no exceptions.

At the end of my third year of medical school, I knew I didn't want to be a pathologist looking at dead bodies or analyzing slides all day long. And

I definitely didn't want to be a radiologist, always in dark rooms looking at X-rays or scans. Although I loved the surgeons who taught me as a student, I didn't want to live for the operating room either. I wanted to take care of people, not just treat them and then send them on their way.

I liked adult medicine, and I initially decided to pursue a residency in neurology. I was fascinated by neuroscience, particularly the biology underlying our thoughts and emotions. First, I needed to complete a residency in internal medicine. For that, I chose one of the preeminent teaching hospitals in the U.S. However, my choice also put me on a pathway into one of the most grueling internal medicine residency programs in the country. A program run by a gentleman known in medical circles as "the Don."

4

Parkland Hospital in Dallas, Texas, is a county hospital that also serves as one of the busiest hospitals in America. The majority of patients were poor — black, white, and brown. With Dallas being fairly close to Mexico, there were many Latino immigrants, and the language barrier made practicing medicine a challenge.

In addition to being a tremendous teaching program, the internal medicine program at Parkland had one other huge draw. The chairman, Donald Seldin, was one of the true clinical giants of his time. He was one of the last of a dying breed of clinicians who didn't need complicated tests or scans to make a diagnosis.

His mere presence was intimidating, especially to an intern just out of medical school. "The Don," as we came to affectionately call him, could often be heard berating an intern who didn't have an answer to one of his probing questions.

"Here's a dime," he would say in a whiny Brooklyn accent, "Go call your mother. She can take better care of this patient than you."

And he might have been right.

The Don constantly drilled one thing into the heads of his medical residents: the importance of spending time with patients. He compared a doctor to a detective trying to solve a mystery. The more questions you ask, the better you understand the case, and the easier it will be to solve the mystery. Observation is an essential component of this process, he often said. We would learn best by listening. Listening to what the patient — and their families — were telling us. And by observing.

The Don could stand at the doorway to a patient's room, ask a series of questions, listen to the patient, and tell you exactly what was wrong with that individual without having seen a single lab or scan. He used to tell us that we could make a diagnosis ninety percent of the time if we simply took the time to take a good history and perform an extensive physical.

Taking a good history didn't imply a one-way conversation with the doctor asking questions. It meant being an excellent listener. Patients might not know how to use the medical jargon, but they know their body better than any physician. I learned that if I listened carefully, the patient would usually lead me in the right direction.

Today, you can barely get doctors to give you an opinion on your case without first ordering scores of blood tests and scans. It's partly defensive medicine, the reality of living in a litigious society. Doctors often order tests to cover their backside. And frankly, many patients demand tests, thinking that their $10 co-pay entitles them to unlimited testing. Rather than accept that a headache is likely a sinus infection, they request and even insist on an MRI scan. It is convenient to blame physicians for their reliance on tests rather than clinical acumen, but there is plenty of blame to go around.

As part of the debasing experience of an internal medicine residency, I was on call every third night. If I went into the hospital at 6:00 am Monday morning, I might not leave until 10:00 pm Tuesday evening. During that period, I'd be lucky to get one to two hours of sleep.

What does staying up for 36 hours straight do to your bedside manner? For one, you become a bit callous. Maybe numb is a more appropriate term. I had always considered myself a compassionate individual, but I reached the breaking point every now and then during my residency, especially after no sleep and getting an admission at 4:00 am. (When this happened, I knew I probably wouldn't get out of the hospital for another 16 hours.)

I recall falling asleep on patients' beds in the early hours of the morning in the midst of taking a history. I'm not sure I could have endured that level of punishment had I not been young. Still, our code of honor as residents was to never leave the hospital until our patients were medically stable, even if that meant staying longer under less than ideal conditions.

There were weeks when I would log at least 120 hours of time in the hospital. What we endured was brutal. After work, I went running to relieve stress, clocking at least 20 miles most weeks. We spent so many hours in the hospital that it became our de facto social network. The close bonds that developed among medicine residents and the other health care providers in the hospital were life-saving. We sensed we were all in it together.

Near the completion of my internship (the first year of medical residency), I was working in the medical intensive care unit (MICU) one night, a unit in Parkland where only the sickest of the sick were admitted. Patients admitted to the MICU required exquisite attention to every detail of their cases or they would likely die. They were that critically ill.

Some mornings you start to feel that funny buzzing in your head if you haven't slept all night. On one such morning at 4:00 the emergency room called me to pick up my next patient. I'd lost count of the admissions from the previous day and night. This patient had to be terribly sick, otherwise the residents would have held her over for the next day's ICU team that arrived at 6:00 am.

When I walked into the ER, I saw a middle-aged woman who had already been intubated and placed on a ventilator. Her blood pressure was barely detectable despite the powerful medications flowing through her IV. She was an alcoholic with probable end-stage liver disease. Her body was shutting down, organ by organ — and she was all mine. I'd not had a wink of sleep in almost 24 hours.

I remember feeling resentful that someone could neglect herself so badly and deprive me of the only opportunity to get an hour or two of desperately needed sleep. As selfish as that sounds, that's exactly what was going through my mind at the time.

Nevertheless, we brought her to the MICU and started working on her. The pH in her blood (an indicator of the acid/base balance in her body) was so low it was as if she had acid flowing through her veins. She never really stood a chance from the outset. She died shortly after being admitted.

I went to the family waiting room, expecting to find it empty. I couldn't imagine who would be there for this woman. As it turned out, there was one person waiting — a young girl no more than ten years of age. She sat alone, shivering with fear. There were no social workers or priests in the hospital at that hour. I sat down with this fragile child. The woman who had died was her mother. I asked about other relatives, but she shook her head.

Then I told this girl that her mother would not be coming home. As the child wept, I sat with her. I was sleep deprived and had patients to attend to, but I was not going to leave her alone.

"I'm so sorry for your loss," I said.

The girl said nothing. I didn't know what to say either.

We sat together in silence waiting for the sun to rise and the social workers to arrive.

5

Sitting in the waiting room with the girl who'd lost her mother, I realized how dehumanizing the residency experience had become. I had actually been angry with this patient for not allowing me to sleep. How dare she do that! It was as if some stranger had taken control of my body — an intruder created by sleep deprivation, crappy nutrition, and pure stress.

As I left the waiting room, I wondered why there was no one there to help me deal with my feelings and the deep sadness that I felt over the death of this child's mother. My patient was not just another admission, a train wreck of a human being with complete body decay as a consequence of her own volition. She was a mother, loved by her daughter. Who was I to pass judgment? Who was I to get angry because my one opportunity for sleep was ruined?

In many ways, that morning turned out to be a defining moment in my medical career.

Still, the first year of residency continued to be about survival amid physical and emotional torture. I was constantly worrying about a patient's blood glucose level or someone's arrhythmia, rather than having the time to understand the individual. There was little time for that kind of personal attention and even less time to deal with my own emotions. But emotions can be put aside only so long before they demand to be acknowledged.

Shortly after the death of the single mother, a young girl complained of heart palpitations and dizziness starting a day or two prior to being admitted. She had experienced sustained ventricular tachycardia (V-tach), a potentially fatal arrhythmia where the heart beats dangerously out of control. It is the leading cause of out-of-hospital sudden deaths. She was admitted to the MICU where we treated her, rather aggressively, with medications to terminate the V-tach and restore her heart rate to a normal rhythm. What she needed was an implantable cardiac defibrillator, but it had not yet been FDA approved.

This young girl remained fully conscious throughout much of the ordeal, but she was scared to death. Parkland Hospital had world-class cardiologists, and it just so happened that one of the brightest and most experienced cardiology fellows was on call that day. But even he could not control the V-tach. The cardiologist's mounting frustration was obvious, even to the point of tears. As a fledgling doctor, I respected this man immensely. Watching him break down emotionally over the absolute futility of seeing a previously healthy teen fade before our eyes was more than I could take. She died, less than twenty-four hours after being admitted to the hospital.

As the resident, it was my responsibility to tell the family that their daughter would not be coming home. The girl's mother was in shock. She didn't believe me.

"But she needs to come home," the woman said. "She has school tomorrow."

There had been nothing from my years in high school, college, or medical school to teach me how to handle this situation.

I tried to console the family. The mother fell on the floor. The other family members were trying to help her deal with the loss.

I wanted to fall on the floor and cry, too. This girl was not that much younger than me. She was healthy until she probably contracted a viral infection, which led to inflammation of her heart resulting in a life-threatening arrhythmia. It turned out to be uncontrollable and fatal.

I had never witnessed anything like the mother's response. And since I had not been the primary physician caring for this young girl who had died unexpectedly, I felt completely helpless in front of the family.

Instead of being the hero telling them "we saved her life," I was the bearer of the worst possible news. The more I tried to explain what had happened, the more hysterical the mother became. Not only was I not helping the family, I felt like I might break down, too.

As this family wept together, I quietly left the room.

6

As a physician, one of my greatest fears had always been cardiac arrhythmia. The unpredictable nature of the incidents, particularly ventricular tachycardia, was especially frightening because you could seem healthy one minute and be dead the next. There is no time to say goodbye. As a young, avid runner with good health, I knew this was very unlikely to happen to me. Still the fear existed.

I, along with the other residents, was beaten down to the bone with cases like these — variations of which played out in daily episodes of frustration. Survival instincts were in full gear. The stress levels could not have been higher, and yet somehow we survived and became second- and then third-year residents.

The second and third years of residency were more humane. There was finally time to think, read, and become somewhat reflective again. After surviving the onslaught of an internship, where I encountered almost every emergency possible, I began to feel more confident taking care of patients. I slowed down and got to know them as unique individuals with passions, fears, and dreams. I connected with families and began understanding how illness not only transforms patients but also affects their loved ones.

As residents, we served in outpatient clinics where we could follow our patients and observe the long-term physical, emotional, and interpersonal effects of their illness. I delved deeper into my interest in human nature and started feeling more human myself. I remember caring for a morbidly obese woman with severe diabetes, asthma, and hypertension. I knew that if she lost 200 pounds, her medical condition would dramatically improve. However, I sensed that continually harping on how losing weight would help her medically wouldn't have made a difference. So, I chose a different strategy. After getting to know her, I realized that she was a romantic at heart. I promised that if she lost weight, and we set realistic goals, I would buy her a slinky negligee (something she probably could not have afforded on her own) to rekindle romance with her husband. Within a year, she had lost the weight and no longer needed most of her medications.

It was also during my residency that I attended my first memorial for a patient. He was a literary scholar and a private patient of the head of cardiology. A man I came to love as if he were my grandfather. He would bring books for me to read, including a fabulous book on animals when he discovered how much I loved dogs. He told me stories about his fascinating life. He was educated, well read, and a gentle human being.

But he had a bad heart. He had continuously landed in the MICU for heart failure and potentially life-threatening cardiac arrhythmias. Before the widespread use of implantable defibrillators, the only options we had to treat ventricular arrhythmias were horrendous medications that were fraught with their own potentially lethal side effects. Like a tiger stalking its prey, we all knew the arrhythmia would eventually win out. I was devastated when he died of progressive heart failure amid an onslaught of more frequent ventricular arrhythmias.

It would have been easy to skip the memorial service and move on to the next patient. Instead, I went. I felt a deep bond with him and his girlfriend. He was more than just another patient with a bad heart; he was a friend. Losing patients with whom you've formed a personal friendship is terribly painful, but I went back to what drew me to medicine in the first place — the opportunity to forge strong relationships with perfect strangers. Connecting is affirmation that we are all in this life together, although we don't fully understand how and why that connection exists. In reaching out to someone in need, I receive so much back in turn. I learned this from watching my mother.

I grew up in suburban Maryland outside Washington, DC during the

1960s. I watched first hand the social unrest triggered by the Vietnam War and the Civil Rights movement. My mother worked at the former Atomic Energy Commission. To do so, she needed top security clearance.

Both my parents were against the Vietnam War. My mother was one of the original Mothers for Peace. In fact, I remember she came home from a rally and showed us this strange looking necklace with a peace sign — something I had never seen before.

The FBI would take pictures of protestors at anti-war rallies in DC. My mother must have been at the front of the line since the FBI came to our neighbors asking about our family. The FBI was probably concerned because of her security clearance.

After we moved to New Jersey in 1968, my mother and a priest started one of the first shelters for battered women in the state. The shelter was located in Patterson, a crime-ridden, high-poverty urban area. We sometimes received phone calls threatening my mother's life, but she never wavered from her commitment to the women.

My mother used to tell my sister and me, "If you can change one person's life, you have changed the world forever."

For this reason, I view medicine as a noble profession. It affords the chance to make a difference in someone's life when that person needs it most. The beauty is that you don't need to part the Red Sea to change the world; simply reach out to one person in need. Just like my mother used to tell me as a child.

What I didn't realize at the time was that the person who would end up changing the most was me.

7

When I finished my residency in 1986, I chose to pursue a career in medical oncology and hematology. People were not exactly encouraging, saying things like, "That's so depressing," or "Why do you want to deal with people diagnosed with a terminal illness like cancer?" I guess it was a strange choice in some ways, considering oncology was in no way a strong point of my training experience at Parkland. However, I considered oncology the perfect forum to satisfy my need to combine science and the clinic. Parkland had taught me how to be a good clinician. Oncology would provide a means to link advances in the basic sciences to benefit my patients, just as my father's research had led to new treatments for millions of people with hypertension. Medicine was just beginning to make tremendous strides in our understanding of how tumors grow and survive. The role of oncogenes (genes involved in promoting tumor growth) was an exploding area of research, fueling optimism that novel therapies would soon be developed for clinical use that only targeted tumors and not normal cells.

This so-called "magic bullet" approach to cancer therapy would replace the existing "slash and burn" approach to treatment, whereby patients were administered highly toxic chemotherapy drugs with the hope that the tumor cells would die without killing the patient. Everyone has heard horror stories from friends and loved ones of the side effects associated with chemotherapy. Many of my patients told me, and still do to this very day, that the treatment is often worse than the disease itself. I wanted to be part of the coming revolution. I wanted to help usher in effective, yet kinder, cancer therapies directed at the tumor cells.

Cancer is the great equalizer. It does not discriminate between rich and poor, black and white, beautiful and homely, cruel and loving, educated or illiterate. Almost everyone with the diagnosis reaches out for help. Cancer strips away the veneer, the superficialities and facades. As a doctor treating my sickest patients, I have often experienced moments when I felt as if I could almost touch their soul.

Choosing to focus on oncology as the next step in my journey took me to Boston to Massachusetts General Hospital and Dana-Farber Cancer Institute at Harvard Medical School, where I completed my hematology/medical oncology and bone marrow transplant fellowships.

I came away from my residency in Dallas having learned many other valuable lessons, especially a better understanding of what "healing" really means. Physicians are taught that healing means physically curing individuals — eliminating cancer from their bodies, for example. However, I was starting to see that healing does not necessarily mean physically curing someone of his or her disease. Being a healer, which is what every physician should strive to be, can also mean helping someone resolve outstanding conflicts in their lives so that they might live out their remaining time in a state of dignity and peace.

Physicians far too often do not deal effectively with the emotional and spiritual aspects of healing, although they may matter most at the end of someone's life. Physicians tend to avoid these areas because they require time, something many physicians don't have, and they can't be treated with a prescription. It requires a human touch, which is not necessarily taught in medical school, nor is it something that can be learned from lectures or books.

Instead, physicians are trained to view disease as an enemy that must be defeated, often at all costs. The war-centered vocabulary we have developed in the medical profession reflects this attitude. We are busy "fighting the disease," and our culture has since mainstreamed the idea of waging "the war on cancer." Physicians subconsciously promote the war mindset when talking about "adding drugs to our arsenal" and warning patients when they're diagnosed to prepare for a long battle. No wonder many physicians gauge their own self-worth in terms of a win or a loss. If someone dies, you've lost the war. Losers surely can't be good physicians.

Thankfully, current medical training is somewhat different. For example, physicians are more open to sending patients to hospice earlier in the process. Now, when fellows confer with me about referring a patient to hospice care who is not going to respond well to chemotherapy, I'm reminded of how far we've come because I'm not sure that we were taught to do that. I don't think I knew who the hospice care person was when I was a fellow. At that time, every patient was a new battle, and if you didn't win the battle and cure the patient, you lost.

But is this approach really fair to the physician or the patient? Many physicians have a difficult time with defeat at the hands of the enemy, and they often distance themselves from patients once they realize that they have lost the battle from a purely medical standpoint.

If there is no longer chemotherapy to offer, the alternative response is sometimes, "Why bother?" I was asked many times to take care of people in their last days because their oncologist could no longer bear to do so. I understand that. That's how some oncologists who are in high-stress situations survive burnout. They try to avoid those situations before they arise. It isn't that they are callous (although like any other profession, there are exceptions). Seeing people die is never easy. It affects you as a medical student, a resident, a fellow, and as an experienced attending physician. How we cope with death may change with time and experience, but the death of a human being with whom we've forged bonds does not become any less painful.

Feeling abandoned and often tragically blaming themselves for failing their health care providers, dying patients have sometimes apologized to me for not responding to therapy. What a cruel and inhumane system we've established when dying patients feel guilty that they somehow let their doctor down. I cringe when a doctor describes a case in terms of a patient who "failed therapy." As if the patient didn't want to be cured. The patient didn't fail; the treatments failed the patient.

I wanted physical healing for my patients if at all possible. But if that were not possible, I sought to heal the emotional wounds and address the spiritual concerns surrounding their death. My goal in pursuing oncology was to learn how to be the consummate healer. "Winning" against cancer can include helping people live the best life they can live for whatever time remains. It means giving them a good quality of life and allowing them to reconcile differences, coming to peace with where they are, and helping them transition to the next phase of existence. It's not about raising the flag and saying, "I cured you of your cancer." Yes, that's what we always want to do as physicians, but we also want to make sure that if we can't do that, we don't abandon people because we feel as if we're failures. Being there for patients, even if we can't do anything for them medically, and doing what we can do from a spiritual, emotional, and psychological standpoint is just as important as the chemotherapy prescribed.

In my early years in oncology, every death was exceedingly difficult, and I had to reconcile each one individually. I found it very hard as a young physician (and still do to a large degree) to take a step back from the tragedies that I experienced, go home to eat dinner, and put on a smiling face. I couldn't just shut off my emotions and act happy at the end of a trying day. Oncologists tend to be on the far ends of the emotional spectrum: highs when we cure a patient; lows when a patient dies. Our job requires us to deal with highly charged emotions on a daily basis. We can respond to those feelings in either a healthy, or a pathological way. The way I began internalizing my experiences was not through my GI tract or waking up in the morning with a stiff neck, but instead suffering intense heartaches over patients who passed away because I had invested my heart and soul into each one.

Still, I'm convinced that in the oncology profession, it's better to live through your heart instead of a cerebral perspective when it comes to dealing with patients' emotional adversities. Even as a young doctor, I let people know that I would stay with them every step of the way. At every turn, I assured them they would never be abandoned. It was a privilege to have the opportunity to be involved in people's lives even at their darkest moments. How many others can say they have been in that place for hundreds of people?

I felt as if I were beginning to learn the art of connecting with patients in a way that people recognized as genuine. In dealing with people under the most adverse circumstances, fighting life-threatening diseases, compassion is paramount. And I didn't know any other way to do it.

But I would soon learn that this kind of personal approach came with a price.

8

In contrast to my residency in the inner city of Dallas, the patient population at the Massachusetts General Hospital and Dana-Farber Cancer Institute was different. Most were educated men and women, often in the prime of life, who took good care of their bodies and paid close attention to diet and exercise. Yet they had developed cancer. Many with young children were desperate to stay alive to see their babies take their first steps, hear their first words, attend their high school graduations, dance at their daughter's weddings, and hold a newborn grandchild one day.

They frequently asked me why this had happened to them. Of all people, why did I get cancer? I had no good answers. Many died despite receiving the most advanced therapies available at the time.

Why them? That was a question that I asked in my prayers, but I never received an answer. Still, as in medical school and residency, there was little attention paid to the emotional toll that cancer and losing patients took on the young physicians.

When I finished my fellowship in Boston in 1989, I stayed on as a junior faculty member at the Dana-Farber Cancer Institute, one of the premier cancer research and clinical institutes in the world. I focused on bone marrow transplantation, specifically regarding people with various forms of leukemia and lymphoma. The work was demanding, both physically and emotionally, since these patients tended to be extremely ill (especially those receiving immunosuppressive therapy so that their bodies would not reject a donor bone marrow transplant). With basically no immune system, they were vulnerable to infection of any kind. My colleagues and I were constantly on our toes, neurotic about every detail, since a patient might look healthy one day and literally be dead the next.

Even so, my fellowship and early faculty years in Boston were not quite as frenetic as my residency had been. I had a good team around me. There were fellows and medical residents serving on the transplant team who looked after the daily odds and ends of patient care. The nursing staff on the transplant service at the Farber was among the most professional, reliable, cooperative, and knowledgeable group with whom I've ever worked. They knew what to do in most situations, leaving me more time to devote to understanding my patients.

A bone marrow transplant is a life-altering procedure because of its inherent short- and long-term risks. In this setting, it was even more difficult to provide the level of care that I believed was conducive to healing. Transplant patients often died or developed complications that affected the quality of their lives. And it wasn't just patients who were affected; the procedure impacted the lives of their loved ones too. The stress associated with the life changes before, during, and after a bone marrow transplant often served to widen any existing fractures in families and relationships. I witnessed marriages break apart as husbands and wives left their spouses in the middle of the transplant process because they couldn't take the pressure anymore.

My official job description involved fifty percent research and fifty percent patient care, but I spent much more than half my time with my patients. I needed to know their tolerance for the transplant, both physically and emotionally.

I remember a patient with multiple myeloma, a cancer of the bone marrow cells. When I first met her in the clinic, she told me that she would have to leave the room if I started giving her "bad news." And that's exactly what she did because her case was a serious one. I talked with her spouse and children instead, who were in tears as I explained that her disease had progressed beyond standard therapy. She would need a bone marrow transplant instead.

Bone marrow transplantation and the high doses of chemotherapy used to wipe out the bone marrow can be a grueling process physically and emotionally. At that time, patients undergoing bone marrow transplantation were admitted to an inpatient isolation room. They could be isolated for anywhere from three to five weeks depending upon how quickly the bone marrows grew back and whether there were complications.

I knew getting her to the point where she could handle the emotional rigors of transplantation was going to be a challenge. Over the ensuing months, I treated her with kid gloves. I spent a lot of time with her during visits. I felt the only chance that I had of bolstering her emotional state was to get to know her as a person. And conversely, she needed to get to know and trust me.

She was Jewish and of the generation where I thought she could appreciate a good Henny Youngman joke, so I interjected healthy doses of Jewish humor (humor being good for whatever ails you) during her visits. Over the course of several months, she eventually allowed me to talk to her about her laboratory results, which was made easier by the fact that she was responding to therapy. As I recall, she had relatively few side effects during the initial pre-transplant treatments. We became friends, talking about our personal highs and lows during visits. We tested new jokes on one another. I remember I once used a Yiddish word out of context (since the only Yiddish I knew was from Jewish humor and the few words I remember my parents saying when they didn't want my sister and me to understand what they were talking about). I think I used the Yiddish word for urinating completely out of context and inappropriate for what I really meant. For months afterwards, she would give me a hard time for that faux pas. I remember when she completed the transplant and was being discharged from the hospital.

"I successfully graduated," she said with pride.

She left the hospital a completely different person than when she walked in.

As the attending physician, I understood that healing was a team effort, not the doctor imposing his or her will on the patient. The only time I felt as if I should impose my will was in situations where there was a high probability that patients could be cured of their disease by choosing a particular treatment. In those rare cases, I would let patients know exactly what I would do in their place. Otherwise, in most cases where there was no black and white, only shades of gray, I felt I should provide information so that the patient and his or her family could make the best informed decision possible.

In my judgment, helping someone make an informed decision about highly risky treatment options that could lead to death meant getting to know my patients on a personal level. I could only do so much to heal them. The chemotherapy could only do so much. The rest was dependent upon their mindset and attitude. What were their fears? What was their pain threshold? Was there strong family support? Did they need extra help from family, friends, or clergy? Or were they able to deal with difficult situations on their own? If, for example, from a psychosocial standpoint they were prone to depression, their emotional fragility could have a major impact on the recovery process.

Getting to know my patients and their families required a lot of time and energy, much more than I would have invested had I stuck purely to the facts on the medical chart. I came into the hospital at all hours, including my days off, to meet with family members who were unable to be there during the workweek. I often cried with patients and their loved ones, having become so much a part of their lives that it seemed only natural to express my emotions. It was who I was and how I would have wanted my doctor to be. God forbid I should ever be in their shoes.

Attending funerals was in no way a requirement, but I committed to going. I wanted the patient's family to know that my involvement in their lives meant more to me than simply ordering chemotherapy. A part of me died with each patient's death. In many cases, I had lost a friend.

One such friend was a man in his late thirties named Dan. He had two beautiful young children who were the spitting image of their father. They looked as if they belonged in a children's clothing catalog. One moment, he was a successful businessman with a loving wife who appeared to have it all. The next moment, he was diagnosed with lymphoma. I remember the first time I met with him was in the cafeteria at the Dana-Farber. We talked over coffee instead of scheduling an official exam. I wanted to make sure Dan and his family knew what they were potentially signing up for with a bone marrow transplant.

I came away from that meeting with a very close connection with this man. He called me Doc in a heavy Boston accent, and had he not been my patient, we might have gone out for a beer. We first had to get his disease under control before we could consider a transplant, so we treated him aggressively. When he was ready, he then went through the transplant procedure without incident.

I felt as if I had done something good to return Dan to the person he was again.

A few months later, after receiving a blood transfusion at a Cape Cod hospital for anemia, he began to decline for reasons that were not clear and to this day are still somewhat of a mystery. Instead of feeling better, stronger, Dan started to lose weight. He didn't feel right, and he had no energy. Throughout this ordeal, he remained stoic. Regardless of what treatment I proposed we try in order to save him, he would respond, "Just do it, Doc. I gotta live. I've got my wife and my kids. Do whatever you have to do."

Patients who were in Dan's shoes were often angry — not necessarily because the hospital staff or I did anything wrong, but because they were frustrated at their situation. The easiest and sometimes only way for patients to take out that anger was on other people, since they couldn't really affect the outcome of their own disease. Even when he wasn't feeling that great, Dan was always more concerned about my well-being and how the nurses were holding up. He was even more endearing because he was such a personable, compassionate man who cared about other people in the midst of his own problems.

Despite our efforts, Dan's blood counts dwindled. Then he developed fevers for no apparent reason. And night sweats. He did not look good, but he continued to put up a strong front and stay out of the hospital. He went downhill very quickly afterwards with severe abdominal pains that we just couldn't figure out. I evaluated him in every way I could imagine to no avail.

There was something clearly going on, but I could not put a diagnosis on it despite a battery of tests and consultations with experts in other specialities. When it was clear that he was not going to recover, he told me he needed to go on vacation with his family. After months of suffering, he declined any more treatments and flew with his family to a Caribbean island to enjoy the remaining time he had. The medical side of me wanted him to stay so we could push on, order more tests, and figure this out. I was not ready to give up on the idea of him living a good, long life with his family. However, the human side of me agreed with Dan.

"Go with your family. You've got to live," I said.

A friend of mine happened to share the flight back from Dan's vacation, and he told me how happy he looked on the plane, surrounded by the sun-kissed faces of his kids and wife.

I knew it would be one of the last happy moments with his family. A few weeks later, Dan ended up in the intensive care unit, where they intubated him to help him breathe. He was not expected to live through the day. Doctors usually sedate people when they are intubated because of the discomfort of having a machine breathe for you, but he wanted to be conscious because his wife had not yet arrived at the hospital. As I stood at his bedside and watched the clock, it was clear he was holding on moment to moment until his wife finally arrived. He couldn't speak, but his eyes were full of love for her as she gave him permission to leave. He just nodded as she whispered assurances to him about what a wonderful husband and father he had been.

She stroked his hair and whispered, "It's okay. There's a time to go. And you can go now."

Dan closed his eyes as his head sank into his pillow, and he was gone.

When I attended Dan's memorial service, I was anxious. I halfway expected to walk into the memorial service and hear people say, "There's the doctor who couldn't figure it out. He couldn't save him." But it was just the opposite. His family thanked me for taking care of Dan in a professional, compassionate way. The fact that Dan was able to come to grips with his mortality and enjoy the remainder of his life was a blessing.

Cases like Dan's reinforced how each person is more than a statistic on a graph. Human biology is more complicated than any chapter in a textbook could ever envision. We can never say never when it comes to human biology. Physicians who think that they know everything there is to know about medicine should do us all a favor and seek out a new profession.

Dan's friendship drove home one other hard lesson: I was not going to save everyone.

• • •

My father fought in World War II at D-Day and the Battle of the Bulge. It was only after his death that I found out that he had been in multiple European campaigns during the war. Like so many others from the Greatest Generation who saved the world from tyranny, he didn't talk about it much.

When he came home from the war, he sought to improve the lives of others through his research. It wasn't until my biochemistry class in medical school when I read about the synthesis of catecholamines, powerful hormones that regulate heart rate and blood pressure (e.g. adrenaline), that I came across a reference to a seminal article by authors Spector and colleagues showing the rate limiting step in catecholamine synthesis, one of the key findings that led to the development of new drugs (at that time) to combat high blood pressure and a variety of psychiatric diseases.

I remember thinking at the time, that had to be my dad.

When I saw him several days later, I asked him about the research.

"Yes," he said, in his usual way, "we were lucky to make that discovery." Then he changed the subject and asked if I wanted to go to the gym to play indoor handball.

He was a humble man. He would rather play ball with his son than talk about his research accomplishments.

During my elementary school years, our family took trips to Europe every year to accompany my father to scientific meetings. During one such trip to Interlaken Switzerland, an idyllic town in the Swiss Alps, my father and I walked to the river that runs through the center of town connecting two large lakes. I was nine years old. We sat on a bench by the river, on a beautiful sunny summer day. There was a flock of sparrows that would literally dive toward the river in one large group, veer off at the last minute before hitting the water, fly just above the surface, under a bridge, and then head straight up — repeating this ritual over and over, much to our delight. We sat there for what must have been an hour or two watching this spectacle. Though we barely spoke, we laughed together and enjoyed being in the moment with one another.

The joy of being with my father, the man who I respected and tried to emulate more than anyone else in the world, was so rich that I can feel it today.

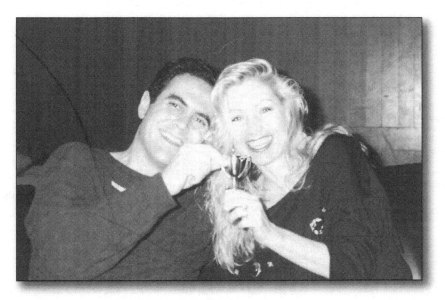

On a date with Denise in Boston, 1991

9

I met Denise in 1989 in the not-so-romantic setting of the outpatient chemotherapy treatment room in the oncology clinic at the Farber where she and I worked. I was in my early thirties, just getting back on my feet after surviving a turbulent relationship, but still hopeful that I would someday find my soul mate. Denise was an extraordinary oncology nurse. In fact, one of the things that attracted me to her was the compassionate care she provided her patients. She stood out as a bright light in what is often a depressing environment.

I didn't know at the time if she was married or not, so I tried casually inquiring about her to our mutual friend and colleague Christine to get some feedback. I felt as if I were back in high school asking someone on a date. I vividly remember the day I finally mustered up the nerve to ask her out. I unceremoniously ushered everyone else out of the lab and locked the door, not wanting others to hear in case she turned me down. Fortunately, she agreed to let me take her out for a drink after work at one of my favorite Irish pubs. I told myself that if she liked Doyles (a no-frills classic Irish pub in Jamaica Plains that served the best fish and chips), it would be a sign. Furthermore, if she liked Black and Tans (a mix of pale and dark beers), a specialty at Doyles, it would be another sign that we were meant to be together.

It turns out that she liked Doyles, but it didn't seem to matter because I later found out that she was resigning from the Dana-Farber, leaving Boston, and moving to Maryland . . . with her boyfriend. She had already lined up another job. We had only gone out as friends a couple of times at this point. Yet I knew there was something special about her, and I couldn't let her leave without letting her know how I felt. I asked her out for dinner, this time taking her to a quaint little romantic place — the kind where they leave the Christmas lights up in May.

I went completely out of my comfort zone, aided by some wine, and made an impassioned plea for her not to move to Maryland. Apparently, the restaurant staff and other diners overheard our conversation, believing that we were a married couple on the verge of separation, given my state of duress. The reality was that we were just friends. She barely knew me outside of the clinic.

Other couples in the restaurant actually stopped by our table and offered their own friendly commentary on what Denise should or should not do. The waitress even announced she was setting me up with her sister if Denise left. When the ticket arrived with "don't leave this man" written in red ink on the bottom, I feared Denise would think I had set up the whole thing. But by the next day, she had decided not to move to Maryland after all, and two years later we were married.

Everything in my life seemed to be working perfectly and I felt an overwhelming sense of joy.

• • •

We left Harvard's Dana-Farber Cancer Institute in Boston in 1993 after I accepted a faculty position 1500 miles south at the Sylvester Comprehensive Cancer Center at the University of Miami School of Medicine. Change can be a positive experience, but it is stressful nonetheless — particularly when it involves leaving behind close friends and familiar surroundings. Working and living in Miami was completely different from Boston. It was culture shock after having lived in Boston for eight years, to suddenly become immersed in the Latin flare of South Florida.

Shortly after moving to Miami, I began experiencing episodes when my heart would suddenly, and for no apparent reason, start beating very fast. The symptoms were vague and insidious at first and made it difficult to discern when they actually started. These episodes lasted less than a minute and everything seemed fine afterwards.

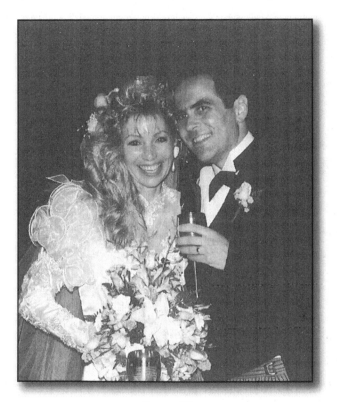

Our wedding

My doctors — and I had outstanding ones — could find nothing wrong with me and did not seem surprised by the heart palpitations. Stress became the most obvious and convenient scapegoat, since I had several potentially stress-producing factors in my life at the time. They believed that the anxiety of adjusting to a new job in a new city was the most likely culprit. Each of my episodes was frightening at the time, but the fact that they were short-lived and completely reversible initially made me believe it probably was not serious.

I could not have been more wrong.

One evening in 1994, Denise and I were driving home like any other evening. We were talking about how much we missed our friends in Boston. I suddenly felt an unfamiliar tightness in my chest, which rapidly escalated to feeling as if an elephant were sitting on me. The pain then began to radiate up into my neck and jaw. This isn't stress. I am having a heart attack, I thought. Denise had changed the subject and was busy telling me about her day when she suddenly noticed that I was sweating profusely. My heart was now racing, and my entire body felt overheated, as if I had just run 10 miles at a fast clip. My blue shirt was soaked in sweat.

"Honey, what's wrong?" Denise asked, putting her hand on my shoulder.

As I described what I was feeling, it was obvious to both of us that I was experiencing every textbook symptom of a heart attack. If that was not bad enough, I was driving 70 miles an hour on I-95, the busiest interstate in South Florida.

I felt an overwhelming sense that I was about to die. As I tried to maneuver through traffic and think where the closest emergency room was, my heart began beating so fast that I thought it might pop out of my chest. I loosened my tie and tightened my grip on the steering wheel, all the while telling Denise how much I loved her and making her promise to tell my parents how much I loved them. I was certain I'd never see the light of day.

As cars darted in and out of the lanes all around me on their commute home, my heart rate became so erratic that I feared I might lose consciousness on the freeway.

Somehow, I managed to reach an exit near a hospital, ending up in an emergency room. By the time I was evaluated, the pain had resolved and my heart rate had slowed. I was reassured my heart was "normal" and told that the terrifying episode had likely been precipitated by stress or possible esophageal spasm, a benign condition where the esophagus goes into spasm, producing chest pains that often mimic cardiac pain.

Stress is without question a major reason for heart palpitations in otherwise healthy individuals and one of the most common causes of premature ventricular contractions (PVCs) in normal hearts. Almost everyone has experienced PVCs at one time or another. We commonly call them skipped beats. They feel like a thud in your chest, followed by a pause that seems to last an eternity. Emotional or physical stressors (e.g., sleep deprivation, caffeine, and fever, to name but a few) can precipitate PVCs. But I was convinced this was definitely something more.

Playing it safe (and perhaps because I was a physician), I was admitted to the hospital for a battery of cardiac tests, including a stress test. All of them were reported as "normal" and I was released.

But my peculiar symptoms did not come to an end. Several days after being discharged, I noticed that my thinking was impaired — as if I was awake, yet staring through a dense fog, unable to focus clearly. The brain fog lasted several weeks. It was so bad that one time I couldn't remember what I had just discussed in a research seminar — just minutes after finishing. Something was definitely wrong, and my instincts shouted this is not normal and this is not about stress.

If the brain fog wasn't strange enough, a few days after being released from the hospital, I felt a strange sensation in my arms when I was at home watching television. I looked down and saw my veins stiffening on both of my forearms. Within a matter of minutes, the hardening of my veins had progressed from my wrists to my elbows. The veins in both of my forearms looked and felt like rigid cords. My body morphed into something unrecognizable right before my eyes.

As with everything else, this unusual symptom occurred without apparent cause. In all my years of practicing medicine, I had never seen stress do this to anyone. I later shared with my physician what had happened, but he had no explanation. Maybe it was a delayed inflammatory reaction to having had an intravenous catheter in my arm during the hospitalization, he theorized. Maybe. But I wondered if I was really so unlucky to have such bizarre symptoms occurring independently of one another, or could they somehow be tied together?

As a teenager, I had experienced supraventricular tachycardia (SVT), a cardiac arrhythmia sometimes seen in healthy young people with normal hearts. SVT is generally precipitated by exertion, which in my case was the strenuous exercise I performed when I played sports in school.

The palpitations I was now experiencing had completely different qualities than those of SVT. First, they lasted only a matter of seconds, whereas the SVT could last 30 minutes or more until terminated with medication. Second, the palpitations brought with them a terrifying sense of impending doom, which I had never felt with SVT. Finally, where my episodes of SVT had always followed strenuous exercise, the palpitations I experienced were completely unpredictable. They might arise while driving, reading, watching television, eating, or simply resting in bed.

Despite my growing concern about my health, I continued to see patients, saying nothing about my problems to anyone other than Denise and my doctor. More blood tests followed, all with negative results. My internist was becoming frustrated and concerned over the persistent nature of my symptoms. Still, he had no answers.

Next, I began having extended episodes of bradycardia (a slow heart rate typically less than 60 beats per minute). Sometimes my heart rate would slow to only 35-40 beats per minute for days to weeks at a time. If I were still actively running marathons or was a professional athlete, a remarkably slow heart rate would just be a reflection of excellent cardiorespiratory conditioning. But I had not been running and I was not an elite athlete. However, as mysteriously as it occurred, the bradycardia spontaneously resolved. And after several weeks, the brain fog finally lifted without intervention.

I was confused. Should I believe a team of doctors assuring me that nothing was wrong? Or follow my gut instinct exhorting me to unearth the mystery responsible for my downwardly spiraling health?

I was beginning to question my sanity.

10

I remembered a Greek legend. One that illustrated the torment of tragedy being thinly restrained by chance. In the story, Damocles was a courtier who envied the royal position of a tyrant king named Dionysius. To teach him a lesson, one day Dionysius offered to trade positions with Damocles, who readily accepted, looking forward to being pampered by all the luxuries afforded a king. But Dionysius had also arranged for a huge sword to hang above the throne, secured only by a single hair of a horse's tail. In the end, Damocles begged Dionysius to switch places because he could no longer bear the anxiety of knowing he could die at any moment.

I was trying to carve out an ordinary life, but I felt like Damocles with a sword constantly hanging over my head. I found my mind bombarded by a silent, running commentary that I could neither trust nor control.

• • •

Your gut instinct is not a stomachache. I consider it akin to your soul communicating with you. If your gut instinct makes you feel uneasy about something, especially your health, take notice.

In my experience, many patients dismiss their instincts because they are either enamored by a physician or they're intimidated by the medical profession. Patients may not be able to put their finger on why they feel uneasy about their health condition, despite the assurances they have received from their doctor that nothing's wrong. It is likely they don't know the medical terminology for their symptoms; however, their gut instinct is telling them that something is definitely wrong. Sometimes, it may be telling them not to accept a diagnosis they have been given.

During one of my lingering episodes of bradycardia, I managed to see a cardiologist who performed another stress test to determine whether my heart rate would increase appropriately in response to exercise. It did, which left him confused as to why I was experiencing episodes of slow heart rate.

"The symptoms might be completely innocuous," he said, "or they might represent a harbinger of something bad." Then he took a deep breath, "It is possible your symptoms could worsen and you might need a permanent heart pacemaker someday."

I was an otherwise healthy man in his thirties. I still exercised regularly. It seemed impossible to comprehend. A pacemaker?

The doctor recommended that I continue to exercise and not adjust any of my activities. Again, stress was introduced as a likely cause of my trouble. I couldn't help but wonder how stress could be responsible for my symptoms when during the most demanding years of my life I had never experienced cardiac arrhythmias. I had often worked over 120 hours a week during my three years of residency, under demanding conditions. I was responsible for the care of severely ill people whose lives hung in the balance of my every decision — generally following 48 hours of sleep deprivation. During all that time, I'd never experienced cardiac symptoms. Every instinct told me: there had to be something else.

My cousin Steven had multiple sclerosis (MS) for decades. As a young man before his diagnosis, he complained of sweaty palms and other vague symptoms. At the time, he was told his symptoms were most likely psychological in origin. As it turned out, his symptoms were probably the first signs of MS. How many people seeking medical relief from vague, neurological complaints are advised not to worry because their symptoms appear to be stress-related? And yet they are diagnosed months to years later with multiple sclerosis. In the interim, they have suffered permanent neurological damage. Had they been appropriately diagnosed earlier, could their fate have been avoided?

And what about the thousands of people with autoimmune diseases such as rheumatoid arthritis and lupus who slip through the cracks of the medical system because their symptoms do not fit a pattern recognizable to most physicians? Or, because they lack the requisite blood tests to confirm a diagnosis? These patients often suffer physically and emotionally. They become bitter because the medical system repeatedly fails them by attributing their symptoms to stress or anxiety.

I've found this is particularly problematic for women. The medical profession historically discounts many of their symptoms as manifestations of stress, rather than taking a woman's complaints to heart.

While some would prefer automating the practice of medicine, the stark truth is that each of us is a complex, distinctive individual, so each one of us responds differently to stress and illness. For example, a high fever accompanies a particular infection in some people, while in others it does not. Despite popular belief, there are no simple algorithms to guide the practice of medicine.

In my opinion, the practice of medicine should be viewed more as an art form than an exact science.

I was at a loss for a logical explanation for the problems that plagued me. Unable to give my symptoms a name, I was clueless as to their ultimate course or treatment. Would things remain the same, improve (which seemed more and more unlikely), or even progress? At times, the absence of answers was more frightening than the physical symptoms I experienced.

And it was about to get much worse.

• • •

Throughout this ordeal, I gravitated toward my primary response to stress: physical exercise. In Boston, I had become passionate about running, to the point of obsession. The day the movers were packing our home for the move to Miami, I went for a 10-mile run in 102-degree weather. And I enjoyed it. I don't know if it was the runner's endorphin high I was addicted to, but it was nothing for me to run in the rain or go slogging down the street in six inches of snow. When we worked at the Dana-Farber, Denise and I had an end-of-day ritual where I would run 10 or more miles and end up at the chemotherapy room where she worked. She would give me a towel and fix me a snack (I'm sure I looked beat) before I would shower. I clocked 60-plus miles a week before we moved to Florida. That's how good I felt.

I'll never forget the first time I ran the Boston Marathon. I hadn't adequately prepared for the race and felt as if I couldn't walk for a month afterwards. However, I trained with some other physicians to run a second time in 1992. We were 15 minutes behind the start line in a section designated for non-qualifying runners — mostly other doctors who were there in case of an emergency. The race began outside Boston in a Norman Rockwellesque town called Hopkington and wound its way 26.2 miles into downtown Boston at Copley Square. The other physicians and I took a bus out to Hopkington together, anxiously watching the Boston skyline grow farther away behind us. It was so exhilarating to be part of that community where everyone came out to root for the runners.

After we moved to Miami and with the onset of my strange episodes, I tried to run, but found it difficult due to fatigue and fear of triggering palpatations. Despite my attempt to minimize stress through mild exercise and meditation, the episodic palpitations and highly irregular arrhythmias continued. No matter how hard I searched for an explanation, I could not find one.

Exercise is generally a great escape from stress, but during this period it did not free my mind from anxiety. While running, I had ample time to ponder things, which is exactly what I wanted to avoid. No doubt, there was a lot on my mind. Denise and I had tried desperately to start a family. Like any other couple, we thought pregnancy for us would be a given. About one in six couples in the United States confronts the reality of infertility.

We soon learned we were among them.

11

Infertility is one of the most stressful situations a human being can confront, as only those who have experienced it can fully appreciate. And anxiety is not what anyone needs while trying to conceive. Despite high tech procedures like in vitro fertilization and intracellular sperm injection, the odds were still stacked against us. The physical and emotional trauma of infertility treatments, along with the dim prospect of a live birth, only added to the inherent torment of the whole process.

In vitro fertilization is the ultimate emotional and physical roller coaster ride. I am amazed that anyone can maintain his or her sanity throughout the infertility process. In many respects, the extreme highs and lows associated with infertility treatments probably mimic those experienced by people with bipolar/manic-depressive psychiatric disease. First, the woman must deal with the physical pain of intra-muscular injections of powerful hormones administered daily for weeks at a time. The goal is to stimulate a state of hyper-ovulation whereby multiple eggs are harvested from the ovaries for subsequent fertilization with sperm in a petri dish; hence the term in vitro (outside the body) fertilization. Denise is rather thin, which made the task of finding suitable new sites for her daily injections difficult. Before long, her body was covered with bruises.

If the physical pain wasn't enough, the emotional effects of potent hormones on women can be profound. Studies reveal that infertile women score as high on validated depression tests as those diagnosed with cancer. I have not seen comparable studies to depict the impact of infertility on men, but based on my personal experience, I suspect the average man experiences at least the same level of despair. Unless you are going through the process, it is difficult to comprehend the devastating effect of infertility on both partners.

Denise and I discovered that injections alone do not guarantee the proper maturation of eggs for fertilization. When eggs do not mature, the cycle is terminated. On the other hand, if all goes well and the follicles mature properly, the eggs are harvested and incubated with sperm in a tissue culture dish. At that point you pray. Pray that the technicians in the lab have the magic touch. If you are fortunate to have multiple embryos (signifying that a sperm has fertilized an egg), you proceed to the next stage, when the embryos are placed in the womb. Then you pray that at least one of those is successfully implanted. Ten agonizing days pass between the time that the embryos are implanted and the first pregnancy test, a wait that seemed to us like an eternity. No words can capture the level of anxiety associated with that part of the process.

Questions constantly ran through my head. Is she nauseated enough? If she were pregnant, shouldn't she have more discomfort? After a while, the constant mind chatter nearly drove me crazy. I yearned for a positive attitude but feared setting us up for the heartache of a negative result, which is the most likely outcome. If the blood test was positive, an ultrasound test still had to confirm a viable pregnancy. Even then, the odds of a live birth were slim, as miscarriage rates are high following in vitro fertilization.

Our first attempt at in vitro fertilization in 1994 was successful. Like all proud parents-to-be, I carried pictures of the ultrasound in my wallet. Our daughter was growing, but time became our biggest enemy. If only we could fast-forward our lives nine months.

Shortly after we confirmed the pregnancy, we bought a new house in Miami with room for a growing family. I packed the boxes and managed the move across town because Denise was confined to strict bed rest. The memory of New Year's Day in our new house, dreaming of the future with our daughter Ilana, remains with me today. We sang to her constantly, played music, and bristled with pride every time she moved. In her room, freshly painted yellow with a border of animals, we placed a large rocking chair, where we planned to hold her as we read to her.

From the outset, the pregnancy was complicated. Denise experienced virtually constant vaginal bleeding for which our doctor had no explanation. He only reassured us that things were progressing normally, based on frequent ultrasounds. On top of that, she had episodes of pelvic pain so severe that several times I had to pick her up off the floor, carry her to the car, and race to the emergency room. With each visit to the hospital came the obligatory ultrasound and further reassurance that everything appeared satisfactory. Despite the encouragement, we were concerned that Denise's bleeding and pelvic pain was an omen of things to come. I attempted to conceal my fear out of concern for Denise, all the while realizing she was just as scared.

We finally made it successfully through the first trimester, a period that is believed to be the most critical and the one that carries with it the highest risk of miscarriage. At that point we began to breathe a little easier, thinking that perhaps the worst was behind us. A few days before Valentine's Day, I was working in the yard on a typical beautiful South Florida day just as I had done on so many other occasions. Suddenly, I heard Denise screaming for me to come in the house. I can still hear the absolute terror in her voice. As I entered the bathroom, I saw Denise weeping in a puddle of clear amniotic fluid. After 18 eighteen weeks of pregnancy, her membranes had ruptured prematurely. In a flash, our world had collapsed.

The ensuing seven days in the hospital were torturous, plain and simple. Nurses constantly monitored Ilana's heartbeat using a Doppler machine to amplify it for all of us to hear. It was loud and strong; she was fighting to stay with us. Despite the absence of an intact amniotic sac, the ultrasound showed a normal female fetus.

Our doctor aggressively attempted to save the pregnancy. Denise remained on bed rest and kept her feet elevated while doctors injected saline into the womb to replace the missing amniotic fluid. The saline kept leaking out, so our obstetrician then suggested we try a radical surgical procedure to make the cervix watertight. But the procedure held a potentially life threatening risk of infection for Denise. After considerable soul-searching and prayer, we decided to accept the risks and undergo the procedure.

We were cautious, but optimistic. Just before the procedure, as they wheeled Denise into the room, the umbilical cord prolapsed into the vagina. The pregnancy had to be terminated.

The next eight hours were among the worst of our lives. Denise was induced into labor in the same birthing area of the hospital alongside mothers who were bringing healthy babies into the world. As happy couples rejoiced, I silently prayed that Denise's pain would end, knowing the emotional scars would be a part of our lives forever.

Denise experienced the physical agony of labor and the mental anguish of losing our child at the same time. As Ilana was finally expelled from the womb, ending my wife's physical pain, I felt a measure of relief. And that guilt still plagues me today.

For us, the end of the pregnancy brought far more questions than answers. The autopsy revealed Ilana to be a normal fetus with no congenital or genetic abnormalities or physical defects. One day, we were thrilled about the future of our family, and the next we were utterly devastated.

When I arrived back home and after putting Denise to bed, I noticed that the hospital staff had sent a photograph of Ilana in her blue birthing cap. We had been so distraught, and Denise had been so anesthetized, that neither of us had the chance to hold Ilana, kiss her good-bye, and tell her how much we loved her.

I sobbed, but soon the tears of sorrow turned to rage.

What kind of God would deny two good people a chance to have a family? After fighting for Ilana's life, trying every desperate measure to save our daughter, I cursed at Him.

"God, why are you doing this to us!" I screamed over and over again.

I had long struggled with the concept of a loving, benevolent God in a world where disease, the Holocaust, other genocides, famine, and starvation are commonplace.

On this night, the night when we lost our innocent daughter, I questioned whether God existed at all.

When we wed,
I promised to protect you.
I am powerless now as I hold your hand,
Stroke your forehead as our unborn child is ripped from your womb.
Tears form.
You are so beautiful, even in the sterility of the operating room.
I want to whisk you away,
As if this were a nightmare to awaken from.
You have suffered so much,
Physically and emotionally.
Prodded with needles,
The highs and lows of hormone manipulations.
Why can't I protect you now?

excerpt from "My Wife"

12

After Ilana's death, Denise and I were devoid of happiness or joy.

But it soon dawned on me that the same God I had cursed and questioned had allowed me to stay physically strong and free of arrhythmias during our eighteen weeks of pregnancy. If some stress-related malfunction within my heart was responsible for the palpitations, the fact that it never once manifested during a complicated pregnancy and the loss of a daughter was nothing short of a miracle.

Once the ordeal with the miscarriage ended, the heart palpitations resumed. Each experience was the same, culminating in a visit to the emergency room, only to find that by then my condition had resolved itself.

One day, I was enjoying an early morning while walking our dog when I suddenly fell to my knees. Doctors call it a "drop attack"— it happens without warning. I didn't know what had happened. One minute I was walking, and the next minute I was on the ground.

I knew that something was blatantly wrong with me — and that it seemed to be getting worse — but I still had no answers. And I always left the doctor's office or the ER feeling discounted. When medical professionals would tell me there's nothing really wrong with you, it was not a relief. It was actually one of the worst feelings. I was caught in limbo between what I was being told and what I knew in my heart was the truth.

At some point, we start to question our ability to correctly gauge what's going on within our own body. Everyone else was telling me I was okay, but my gut instinct was giving me entirely different information. It was coming through loud and clear. So, who was right? If my doctor tells me one thing, but I feel another way, someone's got to be right. Either I'm right and their diagnosis is wrong or vice versa.

My intermittent brady- and tachyarrhythmia continued for the next three years until 1997. For those three years, I felt as if I were tumbling down a dark hole of misinformation and misdiagnosis, grasping for whatever light I could find and trying to crawl my way back out.

I didn't know it at the time, but I was finally getting close to an answer.

• • •

In the summer of 1997, I began to experience frightening and strange episodes in the middle of the night. As if in the midst of a pyrotechnic dream, I would suddenly be violently awakened from deep sleep by a loud explosion and brilliant flashes of white light going off in my head. Waking up in a cold sweat with my heart racing, I knew I had reached a new low in my journey. I had never experienced anything like this in my life, and I sought medical attention at once.

The day I visited my doctor's office in July of 1997 remains vividly etched in my mind. I watched from my prone position on the examination table as the electrocardiogram tracing rolled off the machine. There in bold wording was my long-awaited answer: third-degree heart block — a potentially life-threatening cardiac arrhythmia. My first reaction was, that can't be me. That must be the last person who had an ECG. I wanted to believe my reading must be next in the machine. But it was me. That tracing was an undeniable recording of my heart rhythm, or more appropriately, arrhythmia. The ensuing moments in the doctor's office were a surreal blur. Mouths moved, but words were incomprehensible.

After forty-one years of taking for granted that my heart would beat regularly, after propelling me through two Boston marathons and years of running, my heart had suddenly failed me. In a moment, my life had changed forever. The very seat of my soul, as many believe the heart to be, had somehow become dysfunctional. My gut instincts were finally confirmed after years of testing: it was not about stress.

Heart block represents a serious problem with the heart's electrical system. It indicates that something is awry in this amazing process that initiates and then transmits the electrical impulse responsible for a normal heartbeat. As you may recall from your seventh grade science class, the heart is divided into four chambers: two upper chambers (right and left atria) and two highly muscular lower chambers (right and left ventricles). The latter is the muscular force responsible for pumping blood to your lungs and the rest of the body. The synchronized contraction of blood from the atria to the ventricles and then out to the lungs and the rest of the body is a life sustaining chain of events that takes place every second, automatically, without prompting.

Although I was devastated by my diagnosis, it made sense. Complete heart block means that the upper chamber, where the electrical impulse initiates the heartbeat, is disconnected from the lower chamber. If the electrical impulse is blocked, the lower ventricle is left to beat at its own intrinsic rhythm, which is very slow compared to what the upper chamber wants it to be. In fact, my heart rate had become permanently and dangerously slow to a mere forty beats a minute, barely enough to maintain consciousness. The inefficient, asynchronous contraction of the upper and lower chambers of my heart partly explained my fatigue and sluggishness that had become commonplace. Looking back, it was amazing that I was even able to function, much less work full time and do yard work every weekend.

Third-degree heart block explained my slow heart rate, but it is only a symptom of an underlying issue and generally not seen in people with normal hearts. So, what was the problem? It was highly improbable that I had underlying coronary artery disease, one of the main reasons for third-degree heart block in an adult. So why was I experiencing episodes of heart-racing tachycardia? And what about the almost nightly explosive, blinding white light episodes interrupting my sleep?

To address these mysterious issues, I wore a Holter monitor — a small, portable heart rate monitor I donned around my neck for the next few days in an attempt to record any additional arrhythmias. To my surprise, the Holter monitor captured some startling abnormalities, including several prolonged pauses between consecutive heartbeats. Some pauses lasted up to six seconds

— an eternity as far as the body is concerned. During those six seconds, my heart was not pumping blood to my brain or anywhere else for that matter, which created a temporary lack of oxygen (a dangerous condition called anoxia). Miraculously, the episodes occurred infrequently and only at night during sleep. The bursts of intense white light and "explosions" in my head were most likely my brain's reaction to being deprived of oxygen. Had the episodes occurred while I was driving, the results could have been catastrophic.

As if third-degree block and prolonged pauses between beats were not enough, the Holter monitor solved another mystery. In all my ER visits since moving to Miami in 1993, no one had actually captured an episode of V-tach on an ECG. However, the Holter monitor captured multiple episodes of the same potentially deadly arrhythmia I had dreaded as a medical resident. For four years, doctors had told me that the transient palpitations I was experiencing were merely stress-related and nothing to worry about — when, in fact, I could have died instantly from any one of those episodes.

The medical professionals treating me documented so many textbook rhythm disturbances on my heart monitor that the tracings ended up adorning the walls of the cardiology office and served as a teaching aid to students. Winning the award for the most arrhythmias in one human being was not the kind of accolade I wanted. I would have settled for an explanation as to why the electrical system in my heart had suddenly gone haywire. Given these results, I knew immediately that a pacemaker and perhaps an implantable defibrillator was in my future.

The only good news was that the echocardiogram showed the pump function of my heart to be normal. Whatever was responsible for mucking up my heart's electrical system, at that time at least, was not affecting the heart muscle itself. My official diagnosis was idiopathic conduction defect. Idiopathic is a fancy medical wastebasket term for a condition without an identifiable cause. As a physician, I knew the "idiopathic" cases often died. Many times, no underlying cause was ever identified. Doctors can treat obvious symptoms. But without knowing the underlying condition responsible for the symptoms, idiopathic diseases invariably progress, often killing the patient.

Once again, I was given a diagnosis that I didn't accept. I recalled a young woman during my training who came to the emergency room complaining of shortness of breath and tingling around the lips. ER doctors quickly examined her, found nothing obvious, and sent her home, telling her that everything would be all right. They assured her that the most obvious diagnosis for a young woman with tingling around the lips and rapid breathing is hyperventilation due to anxiety. She was discharged from the emergency room and returned a couple of days later, dead. She died of respiratory failure secondary to Guillain-Barré syndrome, an acute neurological emergency characterized by progressive, ascending muscular paralysis, which can eventually cause respiratory failure. This young woman might have believed the doctors when they told her not to worry about her symptoms, but I did not want to suffer a similar outcome.

As a physician-scientist, I am painfully aware of the limitations of modern medicine. Things happen that often defy explanation despite thorough evaluations. Like the rest of us, doctors are fallible. But I still expect my doctors to do everything humanly possible to help. I was hoping they would be staying awake at night thinking about how to solve my case, just as I had done for so many of my patients who were diagnosed as idiopathic mysteries. The sand in the hourglass was running out for me. I needed an explanation, and it was essential that my doctors think creatively.

• • •

Around the time my heart block was diagnosed, I had, unbeknownst to me, lost almost 20 pounds despite a good appetite. I had no reason to suspect anything was amiss with my gastrointestinal tract. My clothes had felt a little looser, but I had no clue that my weight had dropped so dramatically. I had never been overweight, so a 20-pound weight loss was alarming. However, it made sense and was consistent with an underlying systemic disease process that was zapping my energy, robbing me of critical calories, and affecting my heart.

One explanation that came to my mind was Lyme disease, a systemic and potentially life-threatening illness transmitted by ticks. I had no recollection of a tick bite, nor could I recall having anything that looked like the classic bull's eye skin rash associated with Lyme disease. Yet it seemed a reasonable explanation since Lyme disease can affect the heart, even leading to heart block in severe cases. In fact, it is one of the underlying causes of third-degree heart block in a young person without other risks of heart disease. It would also explain the weight loss and constitutional symptoms from which I suffered including fatigue, malaise, fibromyalgia-like pains, and insomnia.

But how could someone living in Florida have Lyme disease when it was predominantly found in the Northeast, upper Midwest and middle Atlantic regions? When I mentioned it to my doctors, they fixated on the fact that Lyme disease was supposedly never seen in Florida. True, it is more common in places like New England, New York, and New Jersey. However, Lyme disease has been identified in 49 states. Diseases travel, as we well know from other examples like the Hanta virus and West Nile virus. The Hanta virus was initially seen in the Southwest, but it quickly arrived in other parts of the country like California, New England, and even South Florida. In one summer, the West Nile virus seemed limited to New York City. The next thing we knew, it was spreading throughout the United States. Birds migrating from endemic areas in the upper Midwest carry infected ticks southward during their winter migration. I understood that we are a mobile society. So are diseases.

Lyme disease can be a latent infection, taking months to years from the time of the initial tick bite until manifestations are full-blown. Since I had spent several years in the Boston area, hiking and jogging in the woods of New England, it seemed reasonable that I might have it. I even went so far as to request that the blood test for Lyme disease be sent to the clinical lab at Yale University Medical Center, thought to be one of the top Lyme disease centers in the United States. My cardiologist in Miami agreed, and we waited for the test results before making a final decision on whether or not to insert a permanent pacemaker. I prayed that an answer to my long sought-after question might finally arrive. Could this treatable infectious disease be the root cause of my troubles? Was I about to stumble onto a solution?

After several agonizing days spent waiting and praying for good news, which for me would have been a positive diagnosis at last, my cardiologist called me with the news.

"Neil," he said, "the blood test was negative for Lyme disease."

He provided no further details.

I only knew that I was about to receive a new body part — a permanent heart pacemaker. After struggling to find the cause of my mystery illness, and grasping at a glimmer of hope that it might be Lyme disease, I was back to square one.

I was idiopathic.

13

I continued to work full time right up until I was admitted to the hospital for the pacemaker procedure. As the attending physician in the bone marrow transplant unit, my professional life was physically and emotionally taxing. My ability to continue working full time in the midst of my debilitating idiopathic disease is a testament to the resilience of the human body.

Although not knowing the reason for my condition caused me considerable unease, in a strange way, I actually looked forward to having the pacemaker implanted. At least it would regulate my heart rate, help restore a sense of well-being, and increase my energy levels. My cardiologists were now convinced that the ventricular tachycardia and prolonged pauses would also resolve with the pacemaker. I, too, remained hopeful.

My pacemaker was a dual chamber atrio-ventricular (AV) type with electrodes inserted into the right atrium and ventricle. This design was supposed to simulate a normal heartbeat. Because I was active, my pacemaker was equipped with a nifty rate responsive sensor, which enabled my heart rate to increase appropriately during exercise.

The insertion of the pacemaker, about the size of a stop watch on the left side of my chest, was uneventful. With the pacemaker in place, I immediately noticed a strange and wonderful sensation. My heart rate was a perfectly normal 70 beats per minute, a phenomenon I had not experienced in some time. It felt great, even if it was battery operated. I spent several days in the hospital under constant monitoring and exercised by walking the halls of the cardiology unit. I was a bit nervous about testing my new pacemaker, like a child wanting to play with a new toy yet not quite sure how to operate it.

Strangely, the medical team recorded a brief episode of ventricular tachycardia while I was in the hospital. That was not supposed to happen. It lasted less than five seconds, but it also surprised my doctors. They decided not to treat me with anti-tachycardia medications but to follow my progress and periodically monitor my heart.

My new pacemaker and my nerves would soon be tested. A close friend of ours, Kim, called shortly after I was discharged from the hospital. I looked at my phone and assumed that Kim and her husband Jon were checking on my progress. Instead, she gave me the shocking news that Jon, who was only thirty at the time, had died suddenly while playing basketball. I was absolutely devastated.

Jon looked like a Greek god. He was fit and athletic with a perfectly chiseled body. But Jon knew something about his heart that few others would have suspected. It was a ticking time bomb.

When young athletes die suddenly on a basketball court or football field, the cause is generally related to hypertrophic cardiomyopathy, a congenital heart condition that predisposes people to potentially fatal ventricular tachyarrhythmia. Without warning, it had taken the life of one of our best friends. Jon looked and acted healthy and never allowed his condition to interfere with his passion for living. He loved life more than anyone else that I knew. Being on the water was his favorite activity, whether boating, deep-sea fishing, or scuba diving. When he was not on the water, he was playing basketball, another activity he loved. Jon was a devoted volunteer in community and church activities and gave total effort to everything he undertook. But most of all, he was a loving husband and father and the best friend anyone could ask for.

Jon had always taken his heart condition seriously, was tracked regularly by cardiologists, and sought referrals at the best medical centers. I had always admired his steadfast determination to live without fear of death. As he had often told me, if he were meant to die young, he wanted to die while playing the best basketball game of his life. That is exactly what happened. He dropped dead during a basketball game, probably from the same arrhythmia

I experienced: ventricular tachycardia that had degenerated to ventricular fibrillation, where the heart is essentially quivering and not pumping blood. On top of grieving terribly over the loss of my close friend, I couldn't help but fear I might suffer a similar fate.

I wrote a poem commemorating Jon's life, which Kim asked me to read at his memorial service. This was not my first foray into poetry; I had begun to write poems throughout our despondency over infertility and miscarriage. Usually not shy when it comes to public speaking, the thought of testing my days-old pacemaker under those stressful circumstances was almost unbearable, but I agreed to do it. On the morning of the memorial service, my anxiety level reached a feverish pitch. I was practically in a panic state. My heart rate was so erratic that I thought it might stop beating altogether.

As I drove to the service, I would later discover that I had experienced a short run of ventricular tachycardia that spontaneously stopped on its own. The sense of impending disaster I experienced sitting in the pew at Jon's funeral only served to fuel my heightened anxiety and already erratic heart rate. There was nothing I could do to calm myself. After what seemed like an eternity, the minister finally called for me to read my poem. Walking slowly to the pulpit, I tried in vain to slow my irregular heart rate and calm down. I probably looked like a condemned prisoner being led to the gallows. At least that's how I felt.

But instead of dropping dead right there on the pulpit, I experienced something completely unexpected. As I cast my eyes upon the packed house of mourners, a sense of calm and loving warmth engulfed my entire body. While only seconds before I had been nearly hysterical, now there was only peace. The shivering from nerves and the release of adrenaline stopped instantly, as if I were wrapped in a warm blanket. I was safe. My heart rate, which minutes before had been precariously erratic, was now slow, regular, and perfectly paced. I proceeded to read the poem without incident and felt completely in control.

I can offer no physiological explanation for the sudden shift from hysteria to total relaxation and a sense of loving warmth. Although there is no way

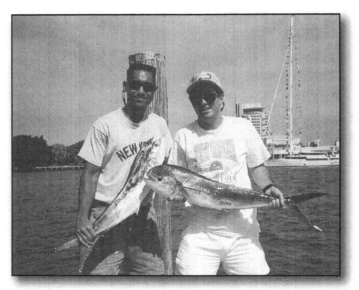

Fishing with my friend Jon

to prove it, I am convinced beyond any reasonable doubt that what happened that morning was no less than a miracle of divine intervention. Never in my entire life had I experienced such peace and serenity. A force more powerful than words can describe was protecting me. I only wish I could have bottled that feeling.

Following Jon's funeral, I tried to regain my strength. Determined to exercise again, I began by walking a mile a day and gradually increased it to several miles. However, something was still very wrong and I continued to feel lousy. I awakened almost hourly, staring at the ceiling. As was the case with my other complaints, physicians informed me that insomnia was a classic sign of depression, probably stemming from adjusting to life with a cardiac condition and permanent pacemaker. Had there not been other symptoms, I might have been able to accept that explanation. But in addition to sleeplessness, I developed such severe pain in both heels that merely touching the sheets of my bed elicited a burning sensation throughout my feet and legs. I also had deep muscle pains in my neck, shoulders, and back. Along with everyone else, I had suffered aches and pains before, but they were generally due to overexertion from working in the yard or carrying something heavy. My pain was not related to activity and was more widespread than anything I had experienced.

Moreover, my inability to gain the weight that I had lost was troubling. It was as if my body was in overdrive, utilizing more calories to maintain itself, similar to a calorie consuming (catabolic) state often associated with malignancy or active infection.

These unexplained problems once more fueled my gut instinct that the underlying cause of my arrhythmias, weight loss, and host of other symptoms had not yet been identified. I prayed for an answer and hoped that it would not come too late. At one of my pacemaker checkups, I expressed my concerns to the doctor, who was one of the top cardiologists in the country. He responded flatly. "Denial is the most common reaction to heart disease among young people your age."

I am sure he was trying to motivate me to move beyond my heart condition and start focusing on life again. But his words had the opposite effect on me. How could my own physician, supposedly my advocate who was looking out for my best interests and safety, dismiss my concerns outright?

One thing I have learned after many years of taking care of patients is that no one, absolutely no one, knows your body better than you do. The worst mistake a patient can ever make is to concede the power over his or her body to a stranger. That is essentially what physicians are — strangers to your body. As I learned from my mentor, the Don at Parkland, a good physician is a great listener. While not all patients can describe their symptoms in medical jargon, a doctor will catch precious gems of information and insight if he or she will just listen. As the Don had said a hundred times, a thorough history and physical examination will reveal the diagnosis most of the time. That is a pretty good percentage, based solely on listening and observing. Unfortunately, physicians are no longer trained to develop their clinical skills. Instead they rely on medical tests, which they often do not understand outside of the interpretation printed on a lab slip.

I don't dispute that computers are probably more accurate than humans at interpreting objective tests. For example, automated pap smears are less prone to error than relying solely on the human eye. However, technology is a small part of clinical medicine and should remain in its proper place. As physicians, we must recapture the knack of piecing together the complex parts of a puzzle, many of which are based on a subjective interpretation of the secrets of the human body.

I fear physicians are rapidly becoming high priced technicians rather than true clinicians. It has become more difficult to make sense of patients' complaints and clinical signs if they don't fit an algorithm. Heaven help the patient whose diagnostic tests do not point to a specific disease. They are likely to end up neglected by the very system that was designed to help them.

I don't believe that physicians' intent is malicious. In today's health care system, where doctors are seeing more patients per hour than is humanly possible, many don't have time to listen. If you don't give a succinct three-bullet-point summary of your symptoms as soon as you walk in the door, there's precious little time to interact with your doctor. The problem is that patients feel intimidated because they may not know how to characterize their symptoms. It's like trying to describe a knocking sound you heard in your car as you stepped on the brakes on the way to work. When I try to describe the problem to a mechanic, it never seems to come out right, and sometimes I feel like an idiot because the best I can do is say it sounded like a metal thingy banging on a rubber thingy and hope he knows what I mean. Doctors can often be dismissive when patients are too vague in describing their symptoms because they're busy, and patients are flustered because they feel intimidated. It's a no-win situation.

I remember a case of a woman who had been admitted to Parkland Hospital for presenting with a fever of unknown origin. As the resident in charge of her care, I spent two weeks performing every test imaginable but could not identify the underlying cause of her fever. Eventually it was time for her to be discharged from the hospital, our having excluded what we believed were the most life-threatening possibilities for the cause of her fever. I remember stopping by her room the night before she was to be discharged. Very stoically, she shared with me her gut feeling that she was going to die before she would ever leave the hospital. She appeared utterly resigned to her fate. She caught me off guard, but I tried to reassure her that everything would be all right. It was only natural to be anxious about going home after a prolonged hospitalization where we were unable to determine the source of fever.

The next morning, I heard a code blue (cardiac arrest) being called over the hospital PA (public announcement) system. It was her room. While waiting for her family to pick her up, she'd gone into cardiac arrest. I remember frantically performing CPR, tears running down my face. She died. Her gut instinct had been absolutely correct.

On another occasion, while on call, I was asked to evaluate a gentleman who also sensed that he was about to die. We thoroughly evaluated him; his blood pressure, pulse, and amount of oxygen in the blood were all normal. There was no reason to believe he was in imminent danger as he had been admitted for a non-life-threatening medical condition. But sure enough, after I left him, he inexplicably died, again consistent with his gut instinct.

Obviously both of these people died from natural causes, most likely a pulmonary embolism (a blot clot that travels to the lungs), which can occur suddenly without warning. People with pulmonary emboli have been known to describe a premonition of their impending doom. These are just a few examples underscoring the power of gut instinct — and why it should be taken seriously regardless of the objective evidence.

• • •

Several weeks after I received my pacemaker, I developed prominent arthritis in my wrists. Due to the swelling and pain, I was unable to lift even the lightest object. As with my other complaints, there was no obvious explanation for this sudden occurrence — no preceding injury or precipitating cause. I happened to have started the antibiotic doxycycline for a completely unrelated problem. Yet to my astonishment, a day or two after starting doxycycline, my wrists improved dramatically and eventually the arthritis resolved completely. Why did a simple antibiotic have such a dramatic effect?

Again my thoughts returned to Lyme disease, since doxycycline is an antibiotic used to treat it. Cardiac rhythm disturbances, arthritis, muscle pains, and weight loss all pointed to Lyme disease. But my test had been interpreted negative. With my survival instincts in full throttle, I began reading everything I possibly could about Lyme disease. I became obsessed with the diagnosis. In my research, I discovered a controversy surrounding the accurate interpretation of tests for Lyme Disease — some that might be relevant to my initial test results.

Could my initial blood test have been misinterpreted?

And if so, I hoped it was not too late.

Emotionless,
Fighting to regain awareness,
Suddenly a Light flickers in the distance.
Pulsating initially,
Gradually transforming into a constant luminescence.
Vague shadowy figures perform their well-rehearsed dance.
Their lips move without ushering sounds.

excerpt from "Syncope"

14

By now I was convinced that Lyme disease might hold the key to understanding what was happening to me. So, I dove into more research. In a matter of weeks, I had probably read more articles on Lyme disease than many of the "experts." I scoured the most reliable and prestigious clinical and scientific journals and discovered many debunked common myths associated with the disease.

One major controversy has to do with diagnostic testing for Lyme. There are two types of blood tests to detect current or prior infection from the bacteria Borrelia burgdorferi that causes Lyme disease. One test is called an ELISA, which stands for enzyme-linked immunosorbent assay. The other test is called a western blot and it helps to confirm results from an ELISA test. After I was told I did not have Lyme disease, I requested written results of my blood tests. Sure enough, the level of antibodies against the bacteria in my blood, as measured by an ELISA test, was abnormally high. This is consistent with an untreated, active infection. However, the second "confirmatory" western blot test did not detect an adequate number of specific proteins associated with an infection to confirm a positive diagnosis, which according to rigid criteria, ruled out a diagnosis of Lyme disease.

My doctors were unaware of the controversy surrounding Lyme disease diagnostics between these two tests and how that might impact my particular situation. They were completely dependent upon the lab's interpretation of the results. The folks who interpreted the results at the laboratory at Yale were unaware that I had signs and symptoms consistent with Lyme disease and simply reported my test as negative for Lyme disease.

I asked that the tests be repeated a second time. This time they were sent to a different lab, equally credible to Yale. Again, my antibody levels were abnormally elevated and this time there were more bacterial proteins detected on the western blot, although once again not sufficient numbers to satisfy the Centers for Disease Control (CDC) guidelines for making a diagnosis of Lyme disease. I was once again informed that the very high antibody levels were a false positive.

During my self-education, I became aware of yet another ongoing controversy between the academic community and private practice physicians that specialized in treating Lyme disease. The argument centered on academicians' claim that physicians in private practice were over-diagnosing Lyme disease and consequently treating people who really didn't have the disease. Community physicians, on the other hand, saw Lyme disease as a valid problem among their patients and criticized academicians for underdiagnosing the disease and not treating people who desperately needed treatment.

Part of the problem was, and still is, the nature of having two tests to diagnose the disease. Most people exposed to Lyme disease produce antibodies to the bacteria, initially a sub-type of antibody referred to as IgM, followed by production of a second type of antibody called IgG. There is some concern that the ELISA test (which looks at the levels of these antibodies in blood) might result in a false positive, particularly when patients are exposed to bacteria other than that causing Lyme disease; their bodies can respond by producing antibodies that may be very similar to those produced in response to Borrelia burgdorferi.

Enter step two of diagnostic testing, a confirmatory western blot, which detects bacterial proteins in the blood. Again, there is concern that any bacteria similar to Borrelia burgdorferi may generate the same false positive results. So, the CDC established guidelines to help physicians determine whether a western blot is truly positive or a false positive. Those guidelines are based on the number of bacterial proteins detected in the blood and the pattern of proteins observed on the western blot.

Many people in the academic community have adopted the CDC guidelines as a Holy Grail for diagnosing Lyme disease. However, medicine is not a black and white world. They have forgotten that the CDC established those criteria to help physicians confirm diagnoses, not to replace assessing a patient in a doctor's office. Ideally, the physician already suspects what's wrong based on a thorough history and physical examination, and the diagnostic tests help to confirm their suspicion.

Unfortunately, too many physicians have lost (or never learned) effective clinical skills, and therefore they are solely dependent upon blood tests to make diagnoses. Most do not even know the sensitivity and specificity of the tests they order, or the limitations of the tests. Instead they rely upon a lab to interpret the results for them. But the personnel in the lab have never seen the patient, so they don't have the full story.

This has become a huge problem. Diagnostic tests are becoming increasingly more complex; consequently, patients feel as if they are treated as a lab value rather than a human being. Oftentimes they are.

My mentors in internal medicine and hematology/medical oncology were true diagnosticians. They did not rely solely on MRI scans or PCR blood tests to make diagnoses. Rather, they listened to what patients had to say and conducted thorough physical examinations. That's not to say that tests are not useful. They can help to confirm diagnoses and, particularly in oncology, select the best therapies for individual patients. However, I still heavily rely on the clinical skills that I developed from years of experience. There is no substitute for experience.

We physicians have to remember that CDC guidelines change as we gain collective experience with a particular disease. Consider AIDS, for example. When I was a medical resident in the early 1980s, the CDC guidelines for AIDS consisted of only several criteria. Today, after two decades of real world experience in dealing with AIDS, those guidelines have blossomed significantly. Had we been dogmatic in our thinking as to what constitutes AIDS based on the original criteria set in the early 1980s, millions of people would have gone undiagnosed, and therefore untreated.

The same is essentially true for the diagnostic criteria established for

Lyme disease. It is inevitable that as we accumulate more experience with a disease, the guidelines for diagnosis will have to be adjusted. Any physician foolish enough to think the current guidelines are set in stone is someone to be avoided, regardless of his or her credentials.

I learned from research published in scientific journals that proteins associated with Lyme disease can vary depending on what part of the country someone lives in. Moreover, immune responses can take time to evolve, so the results from one test may be inadequate to accurately determine what is going on with a particular patient.

Armed with this research, I made the mistake of calling various academic centers noted for their expertise in treating Lyme disease. I discussed my clinical situation and both lab results with several alleged experts in the field. Each had the audacity to make a diagnosis over the phone, based purely on lab tests, and agreed unequivocally that I did not have Lyme disease.

What's more, they categorically claimed they had never seen anyone with Lyme carditis (inflammation of the heart related to Lyme infection) that did not also have the requisite proteins detected on a western blot. Since I did not have them, I did not have Lyme disease, they said. So how did they explain the dramatic improvement in my arthritis after taking doxycycline, an antibiotic commonly used to treat Lyme disease? Easy — that, too, was a "false positive." They pointed to literature showing that some antibiotics have anti-inflammatory properties; therefore, the doxycycline was treating my so-called "rheumatologic condition." Rather than taking an interest in my symptoms, they refused to connect the dots. I should have said "baloney," but I was much too sick at the time to deal with what I was hearing.

I was becoming very depressed and for the first time since my odyssey had begun, started believing them rather than trust my instinct. If you ever describe your symptoms to a physician and he or she tells you "this never happens," do yourself a favor and find another physician. The complexity of human biology disqualifies anyone from making such an audacious statement.

Anything and everything is possible when it comes to the human body.

No one, and I mean no one — even doctors with the loftiest medical credentials — should speak as if they know everything there is to know about human biology, particularly if they are relying heavily on lab tests alone.

Despite possessing classical symptoms of advanced Lyme disease — unexplained third-degree heart block in a young individual without risk factors for heart disease; arthritis (that resolved on doxycycline); weight loss; other symptoms of a systemic disease; a positive ELISA; and two Western blots that appeared to show that my immune response was evolving (with more proteins detected on the second test compared with the first) — I still was not treated for Lyme disease.

Why? Apparently, I was short a protein or two on the western blot needed to confirm a diagnosis, at least in their minds.

As a researcher, I had probably conducted hundreds of western blots over the years. I knew the ins and outs of the test, its strengths and limitations. I wasn't buying the "missing one protein" explanation as to why I did not have Lyme disease. There was too much evidence to the contrary.

As one of the best diagnosticians I had ever known reminded me, "If it walks like a duck, quacks like a duck, and has a beak, it's a duck and not a zebra."

And this duck looked like Lyme disease to me.

15

Despite my instincts and research into the field, I was largely being discounted by the medical community. If this can happen to a physician-scientist with extensive knowledge of medicine, just imagine what is happening to others who lack a medical background. With my illness as yet undiagnosed, and fearful that the proper treatment was not being administered, I became frustrated and discouraged with my own profession. Even my physicians were becoming frustrated over the situation and frustrated with me for continually pushing them to find a diagnosis.

I decided to try to carry on with my life as best I could. I continued to go to work every day, cared for sick bone marrow transplant patients, and continued my cancer research. I avoided telling my patients that I was now very ill, as they had their own problems. I slowly tried to regain my strength through exercise, but it was not easy. Beyond all else, I prayed for a swift answer. If I was not meant to survive this disease, I prayed I would be spared from the further pain and suffering it might yet inflict.

On a lovely evening in October 1997, about two months since my third-degree heart block was discovered and the first pacemaker implanted, while taking my nightly walk just blocks from home, my heart suddenly began to race uncontrollably. I knew in an instant what was happening. I stood frozen in the middle of the street with a potentially fatal arrhythmia, the same one that had probably killed my friend Jon. Unlike the temporary episodes of ventricular tachycardia I had experienced in the past, this one persisted.

It would have been easy to panic, knowing that I might drop to the ground and die at any moment. This was the typical scenario that plays out in streets all over America - young person, previously healthy, drops dead suddenly without advanced warning. Instead of freaking out, I was enveloped by the same calm, peaceful sensation I had experienced at Jon's memorial service. I felt an inconceivable sense of serenity as if someone was assuring me that I would somehow survive to see another day. I made it home, walked into the house, and calmly told Denise that we needed to go the emergency room immediately. For the second time in two months, I could not rationally explain why this peacefulness should pervade at a time when it would be normal to panic. I truly believe it was divine intervention. My Protector, right by my side, was telling me it was not my time to die.

I was at such peace that we decided not to call 911. Instead, we drove to the nearest hospital, much to the amazement of the ER staff. I was rushed to the cardiac procedure room as physicians and nurses scurried about. Despite 20 minutes of sustained ventricular tachycardia at a heart rate of 250 beats per minute, my blood pressure was normal and I was completely alert. The ER doctors were about to shock me with defibrillator paddles when I calmly reminded them that I was fully conscious with a normal blood pressure. Defibrillation was probably not the appropriate treatment.

They then opted to use a bolus (a rapid intravenous infusion) of lidocaine, a powerful drug used to terminate ventricular tachycardia. If you've ever returned home from the dentist feeling like you have a fat lip, you're probably familiar with lidocaine. It's used to numb areas of the body so it doesn't hurt when the doctor sews up a cut on your finger or the dentist fills a cavity. It's a whole different story when it's administered at full strength straight into your vein to terminate VTach.

As an internal medicine resident, I had administered bolus lidocaine many times, but never to a fully conscious patient. One of the side effects of bolus lidocaine is tinnitus (ringing in the ears). What followed was more like a 747 jet engine at full throttle inside my head.

The deafening sound reminded me of a vacation in the Yucatan when Hurricane Gilbert blew through in 1988. I remember lying on the floor of a makeshift shelter, haunted by the terrific roar of the wind howling just outside our window. Within seconds of receiving the intravenous lidocaine, it felt as if the full force of a hurricane were tearing through my ears straight into my brain. I thought I was dying. In fact, I bolted upright from the gurney and said to Denise, "I'm dying!" But if I were facing impending death, it certainly was not the peaceful white light at the end of a tunnel people often describe in near death experiences.

The doctor gently urged me to lie down and said, "You're not dying. It's the medicine."

As he said those words, my heart suddenly paused without an accompanying next beat. I exhaled a heavy breath in anticipation because it seemed as if the bottom had dropped out of my chest. Come on, I prayed, come on. Suddenly, the beat returned at a normal pace. Denise and I exchanged a quick glance.

We knew that I had beaten death once more.

16

The following week was one of the worst of my life. I spent it in the hospital and once again, the vampires descended upon me for a slew of blood tests (none of them included tests for Lyme disease, mind you). All were evaluated and all came back normal.

Next on the list was an electrophysiology study (EP) to address several issues. First, they wanted to identify the location within my heart responsible for initiating the ventricular tachycardia. They inserted multiple catheters into large veins in my groin and neck and threaded them into my heart. The catheters stimulated different sites in the heart to determine whether they could elicit the same pattern of ventricular tachycardia that I had experienced. If so, they would have an electrical road map of my heart and could potentially identify and destroy, using a heat probe, the problematic site. The EP study could also test whether medications might effectively terminate the tachycardia.

In essence, they would come as close to inducing a potentially fatal arrhythmia as possible, while administering medicine in order to stop it from getting to that point.

Despite the risks associated with the procedure, the doctors assured me they were minimal in the controlled setting of the cardiac procedure room. I was lying on a table in the center of the room, surrounded by ECG monitors connected to several electrodes on my heart. As they hoped, the doctors induced episodes of ventricular tachycardia after stimulating several different locations within the ventricular septum (the area separating the right and left ventricles). The team hoped to locate where the electrical malfunction was originating and superheat that specific area, akin to spot welding weak points on steel.

Unfortunately, the attempts to destroy those sites were unsuccessful. Equally disappointing was that the medicine was only marginally effective at terminating the arrhythmias. After promising me that no one had ever died in their EP lab, they ended up shocking my heart several times to break the arrhythmias they had induced. I didn't want to be the first to tarnish their unblemished record. I spent a full day in the EP study, while they stimulated ventricular tachycardia time and time again. To my body, it was like running at marathon pace for a span of 8 hours. I was completely wiped out.

During the entire procedure, I was on a drug that allowed me to talk and respond to commands, but I remembered absolutely nothing. The amnestic (causing temporary amnesia) drug is called Versed. It's the same drug you receive through an IV when you are about to undergo a colonoscopy, waiting in quiet fear for it to begin and then realizing it's already over and you missed the whole thing.

The next day one of the nurses who had been in the EP lab came by my room.

"During the procedure," she said, "you cried out that you couldn't die."

I told her that I had absolutely no memory from the day.

"You said 'I have too many patients I'm helping. Who will take care of them if I die?'"

She patted me on the arm, told me that my words had moved her like no others had in all the years she'd worked in the EP lab, and turned toward the door.

"Wait," I said, "what's your name?"

"Nurse Love," she said. Then she left the room.

She had reminded me of what I believed in the deepest recesses of my mind. Part of me — a part I was not even aware of — knew with certainty that I was not meant to die this way. I had a purpose yet to fulfill.

Nurse Love, I thought. *What an angel.*

• • •

My heart function (the pump function) had been normal that summer when I was first diagnosed with third-degree heart block, but it slightly deteriorated after the EP study in the fall. The doctors reassured me that the drop in function was only a temporary consequence of enduring eight hours of constant episodes of ventricular tachycardia. In the back of my mind, however, I worried that if my yet-to-be-identified illness was now progressing to my heart muscle, I could end up in heart failure.

The day after the EP study, doctors wanted to explore more options. They performed a cardiac catheterization to exclude coronary artery disease as the source of my problems. They also separately obtained a biopsy of my heart tissue. Rupture of the heart was a potentially catastrophic risk for the biopsy, but it was one worth taking in order to find out more information.

The only good news was that my coronary arteries were wide open. Although they performed the biopsy without complication, the results were uninformative. The specimen yielded a few white blood cells, but it was unclear whether their presence in the heart muscle was a reaction to having had multiple catheters placed in my heart or an indication of an active infection. Even after extensive invasive heart testing, there were no definitive answers. I was left with the anguish of a progressive disease for which there was no name and therefore no treatment.

I faced two therapeutic options. I could take anti-arrhythmia medications that had proven to be only marginally effective at stopping the ventricular tachycardia (most with the inherent risk of actually inducing a potentially fatal arrhythmia). Or, I could replace my pacemaker with a combination pacemaker/defibrillator that would provide an electrical shock directly to the heart in the event of ventricular tachycardia. This second option would essentially install a "911 system" inside my chest. A pacemaker by itself only regulates a heart rhythm so that it doesn't drop below a certain rate. It would have no chance against ventricular tachycardia. But a pacemaker with a defibrillator senses abnormal heart rhythms and addresses the arrhythmia by one of two means. First, by speeding up the heart rate, it will try to override the V-tach, so-called anti-tachycardia pacing (ATP). If that fails the defibrillator then shocks the person as many times as it takes to terminate the arrhythmia.

Suddenly, the face of the dying young teenage girl at Parkland suffering from unexplained ventricular arrhythmia came to my mind. Even though ten years had passed, I vividly remembered the terror in her eyes as we repeatedly tried to save her life. After her death, her family had asked so many questions. How could their daughter and sister, who just a few days earlier had been a typical student in high school, die so suddenly and inexplicably? Perhaps she had developed inflammation of the heart muscle as a consequence of a viral infection (viral myocarditis). Or maybe she was genetically susceptible to ventricular tachycardia. We would never know, but what I do know is that her death underscored the frightening reality of cardiac arrhythmias: they are unpredictable and can quickly kill anyone of any age, at any time.

This reality was now an inextricable part of my life at forty-one years of age. Fearing arrhythmias as I did, I knew there was really only one option for me. I left the hospital that day with a new pacemaker, complete with an automatic, implantable cardiac defibrillator. In the event of ventricular tachycardia, the device would deliver 800 volts of electricity directly to my heart. According to the literature, it could also cause contraction of the chest wall, vocal chords, and diaphragm muscle. Among other spontaneous effects, the electrical shocks often caused disorientation, an inability to stand, and involuntary screaming.

It had been surgically inserted directly inside my chest.

17

It had now been four years since my heart problems began in 1993, and I was becoming progressively weaker. The short walk from my office to the hospital required considerable effort and several stops along the way. I had a constant fear that an arrhythmia might trigger my defibrillator at any time. I lived in anticipation of a terrifying, unscripted moment — a moment when the defibrillator would either rescue me, or it would not, and I would die quickly without the opportunity to tell my family how much I loved them. If I got shocked, would I be at work? Would I be driving? Would Denise be with me? And, how would she react?

My life was spiraling out of control at an alarming rate. If you have ever been in a difficult situation and heard the still, small voice from somewhere deep within your soul offering guidance, then you understand that mine was in overdrive. It was exhorting me onward to seek truth and not settle for a diagnosis of an idiopathic condition. Otherwise, I would surely die.

Most people are fearful of the unknown, and death is the great unknown. When I was five or six years old, I used to ask my mother what would happen if I died young — before my parents or grandparents died. My fear was "Who would be in Heaven to take care of me? Wouldn't I be lonely?" I'd never experienced the death of a relative or friend, so I didn't know anyone in Heaven.

My mother provided reassurance. "If you die before we do, you have plenty of relatives in Heaven who will take care of you until we see you again."

I then became obsessed with the image of what my relationship with my parents would be in Heaven. "If I die an old man, and you (my parents) die at a younger age, how can you still be my parents when I will appear older than you in Heaven?" I was very concerned about the practicalities of life in Heaven. I wanted the relationship in Heaven between my parents and me to be exactly as it was at that time in my life — me as their young son. The uncertainty over what life in Heaven would be like frightened me.

Over the past few years, as a practical adult, I'd thought a lot about death again. But this time I was not so afraid.

When I was very ill, I read a lot of books about self-healing, but I read just as many books to try to help me come to grips with my own mortality. I wanted to have as much information as I could about getting healthy, while preparing to die if it came to that instead. Was I completely comfortable with what I thought would happen afterwards if I died on the soccer field one day coaching my daughter's team? In my search for answers, I drew on my religious faith.

I was raised in the Jewish religion. I had my Bar Mitzvah at age 13 and sang in the temple choir from age 13 through my first year or two at UNC Chapel Hill. I no longer affiliated with an organized religion. Instead, I developed a profound sense of spirituality independent of an organized religious affiliation. I believed in God, although in the past, I had struggled with the concept of a loving, benevolent God in a world with so much suffering.

I realized that it doesn't matter whether you believe in Jesus, or Mohammad, or the Buddha, or none of the above, God loves all of us equally. And if Jesus is real, then Jesus will love me, a good person who has devoted his life to helping others, just as he would love devout Christians. In fact, my sister-in-law and her prayer group gave me CDs of Christian music that resonated with me (e.g., *The Healing Rain*).

Hey, if Jesus was real, I thought, 'then please, Jesus, help me overcome my trials and live a healthy life again.' It doesn't matter that I am not Christian; I am happy to embrace the notion that Jesus is all-loving and as such, would love me as well.

So, my spirituality is very personal, not dependent upon a priest, minister, or rabbi to intercede on my behalf. I can talk to God as easily as they can. And I believed that God would listen to me just as He listens to everyone regardless of race, religion, creed, socioeconomic status or sexual orientation.

We are all children of a loving God.

I also developed a strong believe in a life after this life. The soul, that part of us that we rarely (if ever) connect with in the hustle and bustle of our daily lives, is energy. Energy, as physicists have taught us, cannot be destroyed. Energy can change form, but not disappear.

I don't believe in a Heaven where people float on clouds. Instead, I believe the soul, the essence of who we are, persists in another dimension side-by-side with ours, separated by a veil that will hopefully one day be lifted revealing the truth about life and so-called death. This belief in a life after the decay of our mortal bodies helped me deal with my own disease that could have killed me at any given moment. My concern was for my family and the loved ones I would leave behind, rather than what would happen to me.

I now believe that the spirit lives on after the physical body dies. My experiences as an oncologist have only reinforced that belief. I've witnessed hundreds of deaths since my residency, and I've been present at the very moment that people have passed away many times. There's a spiritual aspect to seeing people pass on, especially when they've been struggling from the ravages of their disease. In fairness, I have never seen the spirit rise out of a body. But I have sensed when the spirit is leaving a body. That's the best way I can describe it. I've seen the wave of peace that washes over someone at the moment of physical death. It is intangible, but you can sense the presence of something greater than what our mortal minds are capable of comprehending. Unencumbered by a physical body racked with cancerous growth and deteriorating organ systems, the spirit is free to live on — to move to the next phase of life.

Being privileged to sit at the bedside and hold a dying patient's hand strengthened my belief in a life beyond the limitations of what we can see, feel, touch and smell.

I also picked up dozens of books on philosophical perspectives on the soul and life after death. Some of the bestselling books on death and dying are recollections from people who have claimed they died and came back. I think many of us like to read about near death experiences where people say they found themselves talking among friends or riding on the back of a butterfly in heaven. Whether you accept what they say as true or not, these books are especially comforting to ill people who know they could die at any time. Everyone is curious about death to some degree, and I wanted the same assurance we all want about going to some amazing place if I died. It was a way of reducing the fear of dying somewhere out on the street, alone without my loved ones by my side.

My symptoms worsened and I was too weak to travel and seek medical opinions elsewhere or I would have done so. Instead, I did the next best thing. In late October of 1997, I contacted one of the most respected infectious disease diagnosticians from Beth Israel Deaconess Hospital in Boston. He listened to my story and agreed that a severe case of Lyme disease was not an unreasonable possibility, regardless of the so-called negative test results.

For a third time, I requested blood tests for Lyme disease. Again, they revealed high antibody titers consistent with active Lyme disease. This time, however, after months of searching and fighting the medical system for a diagnosis, the western blot also detected sufficient proteins to confirm a diagnosis. All my prayers for answers . . . had finally been answered.

I had Lyme disease.

A sense of tranquility overwhelms the senses.
The innocence of daybreak is unencumbered by human intervention.
Anything is possible at this moment of rebirth.
Life is rejuvenated.
The sins of yesterday are forgiven without consequence.
As the light penetrates my skin,
Love pervades my very being,
Arising from the depths of my soul.
I experience nurturing warmth.
Tears gently caress my cheeks,
Sheer awe engulfs my consciousness.
Thank you God for the precious gift of dawn,
May I never take it for granted.

excerpt from "The Gift of Dawn"

18

For so many years, I had been told it was "all in my head" when I had suspected for some time I was actually displaying symptoms associated with Lyme disease. I remember staying up all night on Halloween 1997 after getting the news that they finally had a name for my condition that had brought such fear, sickness, and misery. Again, my thoughts returned to the millions of people suffering with conditions that often initially present with vague symptoms. What are they being told every day by their doctors? If you don't fit nicely in a diagnostic category, you are often out of luck. The irony is that this happened to me, a well-trained, academic physician-scientist. I couldn't help but wonder what was happening to the shoe salesperson, the car dealer, or the mailman. Now I could only pray it was not too late for treatment since the degree to which the Lyme disease had affected my heart was more severe than usual.

The doctors now knew that stress was not wholly responsible for my symptoms (something I had known all along). However, I'm willing to concede that stress probably played a role in sensitizing my body, particularly my heart, to the damaging effects of Lyme disease. A few months prior to the diagnosis, Denise and I had attempted in vitro fertilization for a second time. Like the first attempt, initially it was successful, but things went downhill quickly. Several weeks into the pregnancy, Denise had a nightmare in which the fetus had died. Shortly afterward, an ultrasound failed to detect a fetal heartbeat. A mother's instinct had been eerily correct. Once again, our elation turned to devastation. The dead fetus, our son, was removed by a D&C, where the cervix is dilated and the lining of the womb scraped. It is a very painful procedure and, in her case, was further complicated by considerable bleeding.

I had barely begun to grieve for the loss of our second child when one of my favorite patients relapsed with acute myeloid leukemia and died. Lenka was a vibrant young woman in her mid-twenties who passionately dreamed of becoming a teacher and moving her family from Peru to the United States. Her doctors had tried unsuccessfully to get her into remission several times and finally referred her to me for a bone marrow transplant. Before her diagnosis, Lenka had been in the process of relocating her younger sister from Peru to join her in Florida. We didn't know it then, but her sister would become Lenka's bone marrow donor. The transplant was a long shot since her leukemia had been resistant to a variety of chemotherapies. But it was her only chance.

Despite all the physical and emotional rigors associated with a donor transplant, I never once heard Lenka complain. A smile seemed fixed upon her face. There is no doubt in my mind she was another angel sent to remind me that while our bodies may become ravaged by disease, that is not who we are; we are not defined by our bodies or illness.

Lenka was not her leukemia. She was a beautiful soul who happened to reside in a body being decimated by cancer. Although her body was racked with disease and pain, her soul shone through in all its majesty.

The Saturday she died, I had spent the entire day at her bedside holding her hand, trying to comfort her family and praying that she would pass on quickly and peacefully. I hoped her family could be spared the agony of a prolonged deathwatch. Even though Lenka was comatose, and death was inevitable, her family never relinquished hope. They rallied every time her labored breathing temporarily improved. Not until she drew her last breath did they finally accept her death.

At a spiritual level, I believed that Lenka's soul lived on despite her physical death. But as a mortal ruled by my emotions, my heart filled with grief and sadness when she died. Seeing her family's devastation was more than I could bear. When I left her room, I found myself crying in the arms of one of the oncology nurses. No one realized that I cried not only for Lenka's family and their tragic loss but also for Ilana and her brother — our two children whom we would never have the chance to rock in our arms.

A degree of stress can actually be healthy. However, what differentiates healthy stress from pathological stress is the degree to which one has control over the situation. Stressful circumstances over which we have no control are often a recipe for disaster. For some people, stress might manifest itself in the GI tract as irritable bowel, while in others it causes headaches. For several years, I'd had no control over what was happening to me because I had no diagnosis and therefore, there was no specific treatment for the underlying problem. But now that I knew what the problem was, I experienced an initial period of shock.

I'd seen this reaction in my patients after receiving a difficult diagnosis, often accompanied by the timeless and ultimately unanswerable question, "Why me?" Life becomes surreal. You feel trapped in a nightmare but think that at any moment you will awaken to discover everything is as it should be. But you don't wake up because this is not a bad dream.

Unfortunately, disease frequently arises without apparent rhyme or reason, which serves only to heighten our sense of vulnerability. How do we rationalize a healthy nonsmoker without any risk factors suddenly diagnosed with lung cancer? How does that happen? Bad things can and do occur despite our best efforts to prevent them. You can exercise, eat a healthy diet, avoid destructive habits, and drink your glass of red wine for health purposes. However, even with all those practices in place, you might still get heart disease or cancer. That is life, and it is humbling from the standpoint that despite the tremendous advances we have made in biomedical research — and they are impressive — in actuality, we still know very little about the human body and the causes of most non-infectious diseases.

When disease strikes at the prime of life, especially for those without prior health concerns, there is the inevitable loss borne of the realization that we are neither immortal nor invincible. Many of us are taught that education and hard work will stead you well in life, providing a secure income and bringing you contentment and even joy. Marriage and starting a family remain a large part of the American dream, and we simply don't count on a debilitating illness showing up in that picture. When our ordered life shatters, fear rushes in despite our protests that "this wasn't meant to happen" — at least not to us.

I personally believe there are reasons why good and bad things happen in our lives. Our challenge is to find meaning in these events, especially when they are difficult. This is admittedly easier said than done, particularly when bad things happen to children or adults who have done nothing to place themselves at risk of disease in an obvious way. In the movie *The Doctor*, William Hurt plays a physician with an S.O.B. reputation among colleagues and patients due to his unpleasant personality. Suddenly he is faced with cancer, and for the very first time, he sees life as a patient. This revelation transforms him into a kind, compassionate human being.

But I still wasn't sure of the lesson I was supposed to learn from my illness.

For years, I had given everything to supporting the physical and emotional needs of my patients in order to maximize their ability to survive the difficult times ahead that were inherent to bone marrow transplants. Inevitably, my patients would show up to my first consultation with their spouse and adoring young children clinging to their side, frightened they might never see their children reach milestones all parents cherish. After discussing their situation and the nature of bone marrow transplantation, they would look me straight in the eyes and say, "Dr. Spector, my children need me to live." I could see the tears welling up in their eyes before they glanced away in an attempt to hide their fear. I don't know how or why I'd been gifted (or burdened) with an intense degree of empathy, but I felt their despair as if it were my own.

I was on call 24 hours a day, seven days a week for my patients. Anyone could reach me at any time, and they did. I would get calls at all hours of the night, but I never felt my patients were impinging on my life. If there was something I could do, I wanted to try. One young man who had acute myeloid leukemia had a horrendous time with chemotherapy in preparation for a transplant. He had infection after infection, and his wife would call me pleading for help, as I could hear him retching in the background. He did not live far from me, and I would drive over to his high-rise condo in Miami to help calm him down. I couldn't do much to help, but his wife always thanked me for getting him to sleep again as I left to regain what was left of the early morning.

Many times I would be eating dinner out with Denise or having some friends over to watch a game and get a call to visit a patient. By the time I would return, the restaurant would be empty or our guests would be gone. After spending time with someone who is dying, you don't feel like watching the Miami Dolphins anymore.

Some of my patients died, and with each death, a bit of my own heart and soul died, too. I wondered if the emotional stress I'd experienced with my patients may have not only figuratively broken my heart but also may have literally broken it.

Meanwhile, I wrote poetry and poured out heartfelt emotions about facing my own mortality and the challenges of regaining hope. Putting words to paper and expressing my deepest emotions was incredibly therapeutic. "Have faith," I wrote in a poem I entitled *The Challenge of Faith*: "In time, all prayers will be answered."

I sat down and reread all the poems I had written a few years earlier about trying to cope with the frustration, despair, and anguish of not being able to start a family. It frightened me to notice the frequency with which I had referred to my condition as being "heartbroken." I was startled by the powerful evidence of the mind-body connection recorded in the pages of my own journals. It was as if I were experiencing a self-fulfilling prophecy.

Scientific studies have certainly revealed that stress, depression, and despair can bring on or exacerbate several diseases, not the least of which is heart disease. But in my particular case, it seemed obvious to me that the power of the mind-body connection might have predisposed my body to experience such rare and profound cardiac complications of Lyme disease. My mind had repeatedly sent a message to my body that I was heartbroken, and my body had taken that message literally.

In this age of molecular medicine, I'm sure some would argue that I simply have a genetic predisposition for heart problems and, had it been known, it would have predicted the cardiac complications I eventually experienced. Maybe the scientific explanation lies in an overly active immune response to the Lyme infection that turned its destructive forces on my own body. Or perhaps it was an underlying heart defect just waiting for the "right" moment to manifest. I might never know, and it does not really matter.

With all the possible scientific explanations, there is one that I firmly believe contributed to my cardiac complications. All of my feelings of despair over infertility and the heartache of miscarriage, the constant barrage of suffering and death in my oncology practice, and now the Lyme disease, provided just the right synergism to create in reality that which I had projected in poetry.

A broken heart.

How can I comfort you when my own heart is broken?
You put your faith in my hands,
And now your cancer grows.
I look at you and am reminded of the frailty of life.
Once you were healthy and happy.
Now,
The dark rings under your eyes betray your physical and emotional torment.
As I hug you and reassure you that I will be there with you every step of the
way,
I am reminded of my own torment.
Who will be there to hug me?

I have always been there for you.
Holding your hand in times of sorrow,
Hugging you in joyous moments.
All the while crying on the inside,
For my heart is also breaking,
And nobody is there to mend it.

All I can do is comfort you,
Hold you,
Cry with you.
There is nothing more to be done.
I will never abandon you!
Who will be there for me?

excerpt from "Our Pain"

In my dream I cradle you in my arms,
Rocking you gently to sleep.
You yawn, your little hands rubbing your eyes,
Trying in vain to postpone the inevitable, sleep.
As I gaze upon you,
I thank God for His precious gift.
For you see my child,
Birth is indeed a miracle.
One that all too often is taken for granted.

You have two siblings my loved one.
Although they are not here in body,
They will always be with you in spirit.
In the howling of the wind,
The rustling of the leaves,
And in the still silence of the night,
You will hear them.
You see, they want for you what they never had.
A chance to play in the sun,
Swing in the cool breeze,
Or be gently rocked to sleep.
Speak to them and listen,
For they love you.
Yes my child,
You will never be alone.

For now my little one,
You are but a dream that remains elusive.
I promise that I will never abandon you
Until the dream becomes a reality.
For now,
I look forward to sleep,
And the chance to hold you once again.

"A Father's Dream"

19

I discovered the worst part of dealing with a serious illness. It is not necessarily the disease itself but losing control over my life. I had heard that so often from my patients, but I didn't fully understand it until now. As a patient, we become dependent upon someone else (the doctor) to tell us exactly what to do, when, and how to do it. Show up at six o'clock for this test. Take these 15 pills a day on an empty stomach. Don't eat or drink this or that. We want to feel in control of our own destiny, and serious illness strips that away.

I needed to regain that same sense of control over my life that I'd felt when I was seeking answers. After all, I had been the one who pushed for the diagnosis of Lyme disease, not my physicians. But now that I knew what was wrong with me, I wasn't sure what would happen next.

To recapture that sense of empowerment that had been so important, I turned to the one thing that had helped me in the past: self-education. I dove into discovering more about the cardiac complications of Lyme disease. I read about arrhythmias, their cause, precipitating factors, and things I could do without a prescription to reduce their incidence. I studied the risks of electrolyte disturbances that played a role in triggering arrhythmias, in particular potassium and magnesium imbalances. I tried to avoid caffeine and chocolate. I meditated to reduce the levels of stress hormones in my body, avoided overexerting myself, tried to get sufficient sleep, and exercised in the evening when the risk of arrhythmia is lower. All safe, simple steps that allowed me to retake control of my health and my life, and most importantly, avoid the potential side effects of a prescription medication.

I soon discovered that there was not a lot of scientific literature on the cardiac complications of Lyme disease, since it is a rare event. Only five to ten percent of Lyme disease cases involve the heart and it is usually self-limiting and reversible. I interpreted this as plenty of reason to be hopeful, even lucky. The fact that there was a paucity of information on cardiac complications of Lyme disease made statistics fairly worthless. And that was fine with me since I'm not a big fan of statistics. Too many people buy into the statistics associated with their disease. What are the chances that I'll respond to a particular therapy? What are the survival statistics? Oncologists inevitably hear those questions, and I am reluctant to put people into categories. I have seen people beat all the odds, as horrendous as those odds were on paper. For them, the chances of success were one hundred percent.

Since my doctor was unfamiliar and uncomfortable with the nuances of the treatment of Lyme disease, he wanted me to see a Lyme disease specialist. I made an appointment with a rheumatologist in northern New Jersey. She had come highly recommended by someone I knew who suspected that she, too, might have Lyme disease.

I left Miami early one morning in November 1997, heralding the trip as a homecoming of sorts since her office was near Livingston, the town where I had grown up in New Jersey. However, ravaged by disease, I was returning home a shell of the healthy young man who had graduated from Livingston High School in the 1970s.

The waiting room was crowded with people from all over the country. Each patient had a unique horror story of having been misdiagnosed for months or years before discovering the truth. Was Lyme disease really an understated, under-diagnosed epidemic? I was beginning to wonder, given all the people in the waiting room that day.

The doctor's office was clearly a Lyme disease factory where treatment had been transformed into a fine art. She spent considerable time with me (despite the growing crowd in the waiting room) and conducted an extremely thorough history and physical examination. Afterwards, she informed me that she was convinced my Lyme disease had probably gone undiagnosed, and untreated, for years. While there was no way to be certain, she believed the bizarre episodes I had experienced after moving to Miami were probably manifestations of active, untreated Lyme disease. I agreed. She recommended daily treatment of an intravenous (IV) antibiotic for a period of three months. The final month would combine the potent IV antibiotic with a powerful oral antibiotic. For the first time in years, I was moving in a positive, forward direction. Hopefully the aggressive antibiotic therapy would not only stop the infection from progressing but also reverse its devastating effects.

After I saw the doctor, I met with a nutritionist who gave me several pamphlets filled with recommendations for foods and vitamin supplements. I recall that plenty of fish oil, CoQ10 supplements, and a diet rich in protein and fats were high on the recommended list. Then, off I went to the lab for multiple blood and urine tests. I left the office loaded down with huge jugs to collect urine over a 24-hour period in order to test for the continued presence of Borrelia.

The day had been long and tiring, and I was anxious to get home. As the hours into my trip progressed, I grew fatigued. Later that night, walking from dinner with friends to their car felt like a marathon. Dinner had taken longer than expected and traffic was a nightmare as my friends fought to get me to the airport on time. My fatigue began to trigger an alarming number of irregular, skipped heartbeats. The fear of missing my flight fueled the mounting anxiety that something awful was about to happen. I'm certain that the adrenaline pumping through my body only aggravated my condition. Walking into the airport, I experienced an ominous foreboding, and for a brief moment I wondered what I would do if my instincts were correct.

I glanced at my watch and knew I would need to run to make my flight. I had not run in several years, yet that night I was sprinting through the airport, fearful I might miss the flight. In the midst of a crowded concourse, I suddenly felt a frightening sensation that was completely alien to me. In an instant, I was lightheaded and disoriented. Without warning, a huge explosion went off inside my chest, knocking me to the ground. It felt as if a prizefighter had hit me as hard as he could, except throwing the punch from the inside of my chest. I must have cried out as I collapsed on the floor, urine collection jugs and luggage flying in every direction. At the same moment I received that blow, I heard a blast detonate inside my head, too. It was so loud that I was sure the people racing around me to catch their flights had heard it, too.

For the first time, my defibrillator had been activated. A potentially fatal arrhythmia, triggered perhaps by fatigue, anxiety, and the physical exertion of running through the airport had set it off. The electrical discharge and ensuing shock created the sensation of an explosion emanating from within my chest. But more importantly, it had saved my life and returned my heart rate to a normal, paced rhythm.

I would not wish the experience on my worst enemy. We've all seen dozens of TV medical drama episodes when an EMS worker calls, "Clear!" and defibrillator paddles shock the patient back to life. The difference is on television the patient is always unconscious.

It started with a sick feeling like my heart was beating out of control, and then I heard humming in my head — the metallic buzz of the defibrillator charging should have been a warning signal to brace myself. For that split second, not only was I dreading and preparing to be shocked, but in the back of my mind I also knew that it was the only thing standing between living to see another day and dying.

The entire event seemed like an agonizing 20 minute shock. In fact it all occurred in a matter of seconds. Anything longer than that, and I would have been dead. The defibrillator was programmed to deliver a low voltage shock first, followed by a second, higher voltage if the first one didn't do the job. When the first shock arrived, the explosion was deafening. It was so loud in my own head that it was difficult for me to believe no one else could hear it. I had a 911 system built inside of my body. That's about as good as it gets. I didn't have to wait for someone to come running out with the automatic defibrillator or look for the EMS to arrive. I already had what I needed inside my chest.

The incident at Newark airport made me even more sympathetic to people with medical conditions that might make them appear drunk or drugged.

How many times have you wondered about someone walking with a staggered gait or speaking with slurred speech? It would be natural to assume the individual is drunk or drugged when, in fact, they might suffer from multiple sclerosis or Huntington's chorea (degenerative neurological disease).

I am quite sure the vast majority of bystanders who witnessed my first episode in the airport that night probably figured I was stone drunk. Nevertheless, an intensive care nurse in one of the terminal restaurants saw what happened and rushed to my aid. Thank God she was there. Her mere presence and calm explanation as to what was happening quieted my sheer panic. Little did I know the fun was only about to begin that night.

Under no circumstances was I going to spend the evening in a Newark, New Jersey hospital. With the help of several strangers, I struggled to my feet and barely made it to the gate, just in time to join a packed flight (not the prescription for someone already stressed). The flight back to Miami seemed to last forever. It was exceptionally loud with people packed like sardines. My heart continued to beat so erratically that I thought only a miracle would get me home alive. I tried to calm myself with meditation, visualizing pleasant scenes despite my awareness of impending disaster.

When we finally arrived back in Miami, my heart was still racing as I walked off the plane up the ramp to the terminal. Despite my best efforts, my heartbeat accelerated past the point of no return again, though this time I was keenly aware of what was about to happen. I heard the hum of the battery charging in preparation for the next, big discharge. I quickly sat down in a seat near the gate. Even though I had readied myself, I still cried out as the thud exploded from within my chest. I wondered if this was how it would end for me. What if the shocks did not successfully convert the arrhythmia back to a paced rhythm? Was I destined to die in an airport terminal?

Someone called 911 and off I went to another South Florida emergency room. At least I was close to home.

20

Several hours after being released from the ER that morning, I was in my cardiologist's office. He interrogated the defibrillator, retrieving the digital information from the past 24 hours recorded on a computer chip. The defibrillator had sensed two distinct episodes of rapid ventricular tachycardia. Each of them required separate shocks, which were the episodes I had experienced in the airports. He was concerned that this flurry of arrhythmia activity might represent the onset of what he termed a "V-tach storm," which essentially meant that I could be on the verge of experiencing repeated episodes of potentially fatal ventricular arrhythmias over the next few days.

We had planned to go to Nashville, Tennessee to spend the Thanksgiving holiday with my parents, but my doctor did not want me to leave town. He believed that I needed careful monitoring. I insisted on making the trip to Tennessee anyway because the entire purpose of implanting the defibrillator was to give me the chance to live a normal life. Thankfully, he conferred with the chief of cardiology, who had evaluated me during my initial admission to the hospital several months earlier. He agreed that I should spend the holiday with my parents and affirmed my desire to live as normal a life as possible.

Before we left for Nashville, I had a special intravenous catheter, called a PICC line, inserted in my right forearm. For the next three months it would be the portal through which I would receive potent antibiotics to treat the Lyme disease. From the outset, I wondered how I would tolerate these daily injections. Even the most innocuous course of oral antibiotics for bronchitis or strep throat had always created havoc in my gut. My anxiety about starting an aggressive antibiotic regimen only served to fuel the mounting tension. My body did not get along with the new nightly routine. Within moments following my first injection, I shook uncontrollably and felt dizzy and light-headed. The reaction lasted at least an hour. Denise and I wondered if we could make it through three months of this.

If I were having an allergic reaction, we knew to call emergency services. But my breathing was not labored, so we agreed that it could not be too serious. As a safeguard against a reaction, I took an antihistamine. Thankfully, the episode resolved without dire consequence. As we found out later, the reaction was caused as the dying bacteria killed by the antibiotic released toxic substances into the bloodstream — a Jarisch-Hersheimer reaction, not uncommon in Lyme disease sufferers treated with a first dose of antibiotics. Denise and I left for Nashville several days later. I was so weak that I required a wheelchair to get to the gate and another one to take me from the airplane to the terminal baggage claim. My parents were shocked to see their once healthy, active son in such a frail, debilitated state.

We took the antibiotics with us on the trip, and Denise administered a dose each night through my IV while I rested on my parents' sofa. Most people don't realize that heavy-duty antibiotics are extremely difficult on your body. Although you don't lose your hair like you do with some cancer chemotherapeutic drugs, the effect on your energy level can be just as pronounced. As the drug coursed through my veins, I once more tried to visualize a tranquil, tropical scene, though that image was far removed from reality.

That entire Thanksgiving holiday was a blur. I was barely able to get up from the couch. My energy was gone. Walking to the bathroom required major effort. At one point, I foolishly attempted to walk around the block with my father, figuring a little exercise would improve my situation. But it had the opposite effect. I could barely get out the front door.

After months of awaiting a definitive diagnosis — and then finally getting one — I began to doubt whether I would live long enough to benefit from the treatment.

• • •

I've learned in my career that the cure is often worse than the disease.

Three months of high dose, intravenous antibiotics exacted a heavy toll. I was tired constantly. I had no appetite. I was emotionally drained. Having suffered from a serious infection that had gone untreated for years, coupled with the powerful antibiotics, it seemed natural at first to feel exhausted. And by exhausted, I mean that I had absolutely no energy, not one iota.

Fortunately, I discovered acidophilus pills at a local health food store, a lifesaver for someone facing a long or intense course of antibiotics. Since antibiotics kill the good bacteria along with the bad, acidophilus replaces the normal bacteria residing in the GI tract that protect us from pathogens and havoc on the intestines.

At work, I received my intravenous antibiotics in the chemotherapy infusion room down the hall from my office at the cancer center. I sat quietly next to patients, some of them my patients, who were undergoing chemotherapy treatment. They looked at me with a sympathetic look on their faces. Without speaking a word, the message was clear, we were all in the same boat, trying to make the best of a less than ideal situation. After each treatment, I would roll down my sleeve and return to my office.

The last month of treatment finally arrived and it was particularly brutal. In addition to my daily dose of intravenous antibiotic, I also took a powerful oral antibiotic each day for the entire month. I noticed that I no longer experienced arthritis, insomnia, or the burning sensation on the soles of my feet. However, my heart block persisted, a rather unusual occurrence for cardiac complications related to Lyme disease since they typically reverse with antibiotics. Since my infection had gone untreated for several years, the worst possibility was that sufficient time had passed for the infection to cause permanent damage to the electrical system in my heart. Yet I remained hopeful because many of the other bizarre symptoms that had plagued me before treatment had completely resolved. Where there is life, there's hope, and I didn't give up believing that my heart might recover as well.

When my treatment was over, I planned to focus on my emotional and spiritual healing. But I knew my physical recovery would be a very slow process, even though exercise had been the lifeblood of my existence. It had been a long time since I had engaged in the level of physical activity I had always enjoyed.

My first step was to start slowly. I relegated myself to walking on the Nordic Track for a few minutes a day and barely broke a sweat. I wasn't short of breath, but I felt limited by sheer fatigue. Even something as innocuous as giving a lecture was taxing, which essentially required standing in front of an audience and talking for 45 minutes.

I assumed that my level of energy would improve with tincture of time. I could wait it out. I was embracing patience. And why not be optimistic? Antibiotic therapies like mine had a proven track record of successfully treating the disease. The research showed that even when rare heart complications did occur with Lyme disease, they were nearly always reversible. Everyone I talked to reassured me that heart block requiring a permanent pacemaker was a very rare complication.

Be patient, it is bound to get better, I told myself. But I fought dark thoughts lurking in the back of my mind that my problems were far from over.

As the weeks passed in the early months of 1998, it became increasingly clear that something was still wrong.

21

On a beautiful spring day, I was walking at a leisurely pace from my office to the hospital when suddenly I experienced a familiar heightened level of anxiety over a skipped heartbeat. Three months had passed since I finished my antibiotic treatment and yet I had continued having frequent arrhythmias. I took a few more steps and felt a flurry of irregular heartbeats. Shouldn't my heart be healed by now? I thought as I quickly took a seat on a nearby bench.

The heavy sensation in your chest and the long pause that follows a premature ventricular contraction is an unforgettable sensation, especially when it happens repeatedly every hour. It can take your breath away waiting for the next beat. Each skipped beat underscored the precarious nature of my existence. It became a blatant reminder that whatever damage had already occurred to my heart might not be reversible after all. Would I be alive in six months? Would the next skipped beat be the one that would take my life?

It was around that time that I began having a recurring dream, a rather pleasant one at that. In the dream, my cardiologist would stroll into the examination room and exuberantly proclaim, "Congratulations, the antibiotics worked! You no longer need a pacemaker/defibrillator!" Upon awakening, I could imagine, if only for a fleeting instance, that my heart was whole again. But my dreams of having it removed now seemed just that: distant, unattainable fantasy.

My family, friends and colleagues did their best to keep me from getting discouraged over the slow pace of my recovery.

Be patient, I kept repeating.

Lyme disease wasn't like strep throat, where ten days of antibiotics clears the infection. Complications of Lyme disease, particularly those involving the heart, could take years to resolve. As a famous infectious disease expert had told me at the time of my diagnosis, if I'd had the condition for several years before it was diagnosed and properly treated, it could take twice as many years to completely resolve. Nine months had passed with no resolution of the heart block or frequent arrhythmias. As the days and weeks progressed, I became more anxious. I feared I had reached a plateau in my recovery.

During the spring of 1998, I had this strange sensation as if my heart were a rubber band, wound tight and ready to uncoil at any moment. Maybe it was my imagination, but that sensation seemed to precede the onset of skipped beats. Rather pedestrian movements, like stretching to reach for a glass on a top shelf, would precipitate the uncoiling of the rubber band. I hated the sensation because it ushered in a flurry of skipped beats along with a sick feeling as if I were overdosing on adrenaline.

After struggling to stay alive during the months and years prior to my diagnosis, a new and equally formidable challenge had now emerged: living with the constant anxiety of knowing a lethal arrhythmia might be just around the corner. There was simply no way to know what was going to be a harmless skipped beat and what might trigger a chain of events culminating in my death.

The defibrillator was like living with a ticking time bomb in my chest with no way to know when or where it might explode. I became neurotic, never knowing which skipped beat would activate the defibrillator and deliver a shock to my heart. I could be driving 70 miles an hour on a highway and all of a sudden experience a lightheaded, weird feeling in my head and chest. With only seconds to pull over, I would brace myself and prepare for the worst. I often prayed that I wouldn't pass out or get shocked while I was driving.

The experience of being shocked not only becomes etched in your mind but also remains imprinted in every cell in the body, making it nearly impossible to forget. Ironically, the physiologic consequences of living in constant fear and stress, and the increased levels of adrenaline, probably served to trigger more skipped beats. It became a vicious cycle: fear of arrhythmias triggering more arrhythmias. If fear alone was not the culprit, it certainly was not helping the situation.

I began to purposefully avoid certain movements, paranoid that they would trigger an arrhythmia. I was grasping for straws and willing to do anything to get my life back on track. There were precious few moments during the day when I wasn't checking my pulse. I obsessed over every heartbeat.

Sometimes I would convince myself that my heart was racing wildly out of control, when in fact it might only be beating 88 times per minute, a normal rate. I was used to a fixed heart rate of 70 beats per minute (due to the constant rhythm of the pacemaker) so even a small increase felt dangerous. All I wanted to do was to awaken from this nightmare to find that everything was back to normal.

I became a slave to my heart.

It was a frighteningly familiar fear that I had seen during my residency in patients with serious ventricular arrhythmias. They had an all-consuming anxiety that comes with the knowledge that you might drop dead at any given moment without the slightest hint as to when or where it might occur. If an arrhythmia struck, all they could do was try to get help quickly before losing consciousness.

Among my fellow doctors, these patients were referred to as "cardiac cripples" — individuals who simply could not move beyond their fear of dying from a sudden cardiac event. (The term was a misnomer since these folks were not physically impaired, just emotional train wrecks.) Some had already been to the brink of death, requiring CPR. They feared exercise, sex, or any activity that would increase their heart rate and possibly precipitate a sudden arrhythmia. Their fear was often so intense that it forced them to become recluses, preferring the security of familiar surroundings rather than risk venturing outside.

Although I was sympathetic as a young resident then, I'd had a difficult time truly understanding how these men and women could live under the threat of constant peril.

Now I was living it. And once again, I felt like Damocles.

What if an arrhythmia strikes while I'm driving? What if it happens when I'm swimming and I drown? What if my defibrillator malfunctions? Would I simply keel over and die sitting at my desk? Would I drop dead in the middle of a conversation with a colleague?

What if I feel dizzy or sense the onset of a rapid rhythm . . . should I call 911 immediately? Or maybe wait to see if my defibrillator kicked in? I can't call 911 every time I feel a flurry of skipped beats. But what if I decided not to call and the defibrillator didn't work properly?

Would it be too late to call for help?

Would I even be conscious to call at all?

Getting beyond my fears would not be easy. The first task at hand was to cut off the internal conversation.

After struggling for months after the diagnosis of Lyme disease, I reached the breaking point. I was faced with a critical choice. Would I live the remainder of my life — whether that might be five days, five months, or 50 years — in constant fear? Or would I be able to regain some semblance of control and proceed to live as best I could?

I recalled the words of a close friend and cancer survivor, Mort Silverblatt. "Neil, take one day at a time and live each one as if it was your last," he told me. "That's all any of us can do."

And that's exactly what I decided to do.

Find solace in self-reflection,
Where the truth of eternal life will be manifest.
Fear is negative,
A destructive force created by the physical mind
To protect the Ego from the omnipotent Soul.
I am reminded,
"Love yourself, for within each of us lies the essence of Divine Light."
Seek the Light,
And you will never fear again."

As I reflect on the moment,
A sense of calm envelops my very being.
Even the mind,
Creator of my fears,
Understands the true purpose of my existence.
Love always,
Have faith.
Embrace life!

excerpt from "Fighting Back"

22

One morning while I was shaving I stopped and took a long look in the mirror. I could see something or someone staring back at me, and it was more than just tired flesh. Behind the brown eyes, I met the arresting stare of an undaunted spirit and soul, seemingly testing my resilience. Did I want to look back on my life and only remember fear and negativity? What a miserable existence that would be. I had wasted too much of my life already. I could not continue to allow my life to be dictated by Lyme disease, heart block, or the fear of arrhythmia.

I had allowed myself to be defined by my physical state long enough. These were only physical manifestations and not who I truly was. Our souls are separate from the skin and bones that make up our bodies. It was time for me to fight and figure out how I was going live a full life despite the pain and exhaustion that had become a part of my daily existence. I started reading a lot about spirituality and whether there was a purpose to life's events. I read *When Bad Things Happen to Good People* by Rabbi Harold Kushner. I hoped to finish the book and have an epiphany regarding the black cloud that had descended upon my life. However, there were no miraculous insights, merely the notion that a God who intervened at the earliest signs of something bad about to happen would destroy life as we know it. If I knew that the hand of God would always reach out and protect me from a speeding car, what kind of free will would I have? But the message was clear: there is a God who loves us but who also allows us to create our own destiny, good or bad.

That wasn't very satisfying, especially in light of the hurdles I faced. So I turned to the Old Testament and read the Book of Job, several times, in fact.

I am not a literalist when it comes to the Bible. However, I connected with the protagonist in the story, Job. He was a man who had everything — a loving wife, adoring children, wealth, his health, the respect of his community. And then, out of the blue, he lost it all.

I could relate. I had a great education, trained at the top medical centers, and had married the woman of my dreams. It seemed all too perfect to persist. Just like Job, it all came crashing down — devastating miscarriages after rounds of in vitro fertilization attempts, followed by a mysterious illness that was wreaking havoc physically and emotionally. And yet, unlike Job, there were times that I did curse God for what He had "done to us."

Job taught me a lesson. We have to trust in the Lord, for the world of the divine is beyond our grasp. I slowly began to lose the anger, and once again began to trust in God. I began to reaffirm my prior belief that there is a grand plan, which we as mortal human beings are not privy to.

About the same time, I remember a moment when I was praying in the chapel at the Jackson Memorial Hospital in Miami where Denise was hospitalized after the premature rupture of her membranes during the first pregnancy. I was deep in prayer, asking for a miracle. And then a vision came to me. It was as vivid as that day in the chapel.

As I prayed for Denise and our unborn daughter, I saw one of my former patients. She was a young woman whom I really liked. She had died of non-Hodgkin's lymphoma that had recurred after a bone marrow transplant. There she was, in front of me, holding a newborn in her arms, extending them to me as if delivering us the child we so desperately wanted. It was a vision I didn't understand at the time. Denise lost the pregnancy and the next one as well. But I do believe the vision was meant to convey hope that things would work out if we trusted in the good Lord.

That strong sense that God was there, listening to my prayers, helped me through the darkest moments of my journey. Rather than cursing God, I started to thank Him for the beauty in my life. I tried to focus on my blessings — which were plentiful — rather than dwell on the negatives.

· · ·

In 1998, Denise and I were blessed with a baby girl we named Celeste. Her name was a reminder of how God answered our prayer with a celestial gift. The first moment I saw her forced me to face one of the most critical decisions of my life. Would I ease into a life of bitterness and anger over the cards that I had been dealt? Would I allow my memories to be filled with sorrow, the love in my life masked by a cloud of sadness? That would have been more tragic than my heart condition.

Looking at our daughter, I realized that I had to live. I had to see her reach for me from her crib and hear her call me "Dada" for the first time. I wanted to be there for her first steps and to see the joy on her face as she rode her bike for the first time without training wheels. If I ended up living long enough to see those milestones and only remembered the darkness of anguish and bitterness over my heart condition, then I would miss the beauty and blessings in my life. I wanted a life of love. I wanted to experience the warmth that I felt every time I kissed my wife and to rejoice in the realization that I was married to a remarkable woman, my soul mate. I didn't want to die before I was even dead. I wanted to make the most of every moment that I had on this earth. I was not guaranteed the next instant, let alone to-morrow.

Coming to this realization was one thing. Changing my behavior was an-other. It meant directly confronting my most formidable fears: namely, the uncertainty of living in chronic pain and disability. I also had to confront my fear of death.

I had watched some of my terminally ill patients spend their last hours mired in regret and anger, and I understood that. Others became so wrapped up in their disease that they lost sight of who they were inside. "Jane" no longer thought of herself as Jane, loving mother and loyal friend. She was "Jane with breast cancer." "Steve" relinquished his former identity as a busi-nessman and became "Steve — victim of prostate cancer." They defined themselves by their diagnoses.

I was determined not to make those same choices. And I was fortunate

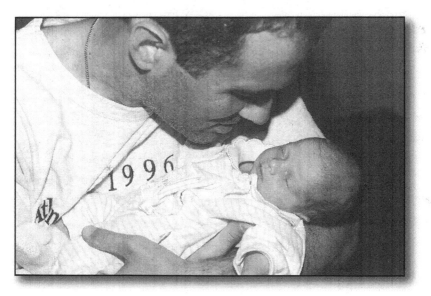

Beautiful Baby Celeste

to have patients who served as role models of courage. I did not want to burden them with my problems, but they often unknowingly guided me through the darkest hours. In the midst of their anguish and physical torment, I saw how bright their spirit shone. They were gracious and loving despite the pain they often experienced, always coming to the clinic with a smile on their faces, more concerned about how I was doing.

These patients, the ones who demonstrated such amazing faith and grace in the face of suffering, are the ones I will never forget. They exuded a love so pure and genuine that it seemed to emanate from the depths of the soul. They had been through trials and tribulations and yet still believed that there was meaning to their lives. I realized once more how incredibly resilient the human spirit is even encased within the confines of a decaying body.

Miguel was one such patient — the quintessential person who loved life. He reminded me of a Latin caricature who would do the flamenco with a stranger in the middle of the street. Whenever something bad would happen to Miguel, his response was just to open up a bottle of red wine, toast his friends, and find something to celebrate. He embraced his life, although it had not been an easy one. As a Cuban national in his late teens, he was involved in the Bay of Pigs fiasco and was arrested and tortured after the failed overthrow of Castro. He eventually came to the U.S., not knowing any English, and worked his way through Harvard to become a writer and director — a real American success story.

I met him when he was diagnosed with chronic myeloid leukemia (in the days before the miraculous treatments we have now). Patients can live a fairly healthy life for years before the disease finally converts to an acute leukemia. When I met him, Miguel was in the chronic phase of the disease. I got to know him well, and he often invited Denise and me to dinner parties at his old Spanish-style home to mark Cuban Independence Day or whatever he felt like celebrating. There was loud Latino music, spicy Cuban food, and lots of dancing. It was easy to forget Miguel had a deadly disease.

One night about 48 hours before he died, he asked me to come over to his house. He had called together various friends and colleagues in the arts industry to come over for dinner to give them instructions about how to complete a documentary he had been working on about Cuban immigration. He knew he would not be there to see it through to the end. There was a spread of food and the wine and laughter poured freely, along with the constant stream of Latin-inspired music floating throughout the house and onto the outdoor patio.

His friends later referred to this night as the Last Supper because he became bedridden and died the next day. I was there for the end, too, reminiscing with friends around his bedside as Miguel lay in a near-comatose state. We were listening to music and talking about each song. A song came on and we remarked that we couldn't figure out the name. All of a sudden, Miguel sat straight up in bed and said matter-of-factly, "Of course, that's Sergio Menendez, 1974." Even on his deathbed, he could pop out of a near-comatose state with a burst of zeal for life — it was surreal. He slowly drifted off again and passed away in the ensuing hours. His life was this incredible celebration, even until the last moment that he could have a memory. Miguel had always said that he wanted to be as awake as possible when he passed on because he wanted to be able to write about his transition to the other side. He wanted to experience the full breadth of the moment.

He proved to me that there is nothing to fear.

How did patients like Miguel and others do that? What was their secret? I did not know for certain, but I knew where I might start finding some answers. In order to move ahead with my life, I had to settle a question so many of them had asked me in the exam room — Why me? The thought had been running recklessly through my own mind for some time. Most of my patients had every right to wonder why they, of all people, were sick. Like me, these were often the ones who had practiced healthy lifestyles. They did not smoke and they had been physically active. So why did they develop lymphoma, leukemia, breast cancer, or brain tumors? Was it merely bad genetics? Whatever the reason was, it was not readily apparent to them or to me. In my case, my only fault was that a tick had bitten me. Why was I one of the rare oddballs whose cardiac complications had not reversed with antibiotics? Why was I now the owner of a permanent pacemaker/defibrillator? Maybe the answer was something my grandmother used to say: "Why not you?"

Western medicine is limited when it comes to answering the "why me" question. We have become very good at treating symptoms, but our ability to cure the underlying medical condition leaves a lot to be desired. For example, we never cure hypertension since we really don't know its etiology. We can manage it primarily with medications (although diet and lifestyle changes are recognized as important aspects of treatment as well). My pacemaker/defibrillator was managing the electrical disturbance in my heart, but it clearly wasn't going to heal it. I would have to take matters into my own hands.

In the absence of understanding why their disease happened to them, many of my patients turned to spirituality for comfort. Knowing that there is a higher power and recognizing that there is order to the universe provided them with a sense of solace. In the end, I realized that maybe it isn't important to have a definite answer to the question. The answer is beyond my comprehension anyway.

Instead of wanting to know why this had happened, I now began focusing on what I was going to do about it.

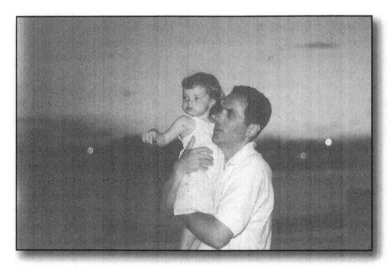

Celeste and me

Have faith I am told.
Like the swallows returning to Capistrano
Good fortune will surely come your way.
Have faith.
When nature deals a cruel hand,
Have faith,
Lest you forget that nature is also beauty, joy, and love.
When you have looked into the abyss and seen no escape,
Have faith,
For light will illuminate even the most impenetrable recesses of the mind.
When your thoughts center on doubt and uncertainties.
Have faith,
Listen quietly, for the still small voice heralds peace and harmony.
When your legs can move no further,
And your body is racked with pain.
Have faith,
Allow the universal energy to flow within your body,
Rejuvenating the weary spirit.
When mere mortals insist that your dreams are impossible,
Have faith,
Open your eyes and witness the miracles of life.
Everything is possible to the faithful.
In good time all prayers will be answered.

excerpt from "The Challenge of Faith"

23

Heal *def.*: to make whole or sound
Merriam-Webster Dictionary

Healing is a process that ultimately comes from within.

I am not talking about recovering from an episode of laryngitis; in that case, we don't need to meditate on the meaning of life. However, after being diagnosed with a serious chronic medical or psychiatric condition, rendering ourselves whole is difficult. Add to that the daunting realization that we'll have to deal with the consequences of the disease for the rest of our lives. I needed physical and emotional healing. I tried to be the best patient I could possibly be, not only doing what I needed to do from the standpoint of western medicine (medication), but also (and perhaps more importantly) doing what was under my control to maintain my emotional well-being. My slow return to exercise was helping me to regain my physical health. Gradually, the physical pain subsided. My endurance slowly increased. For the first time in months, I felt alive, as if my life was returning to some semblance of normalcy. I was thinking more clearly. I realized that I could exercise without triggering arrhythmias. I was reclaiming a small piece of what had once been the cornerstone of my life.

But how could I become whole again? Exercise, diet, and nutritional supplements were certainly important components to healing, particularly to restoring physical well-being, but they did not necessarily lead to emotional healing. I believe in the mind-body connection. I began to work on healing something the medical profession often neglects: my mind.

Although I had meditated intermittently over the years, I began to meditate on a daily basis with a sense of purpose. Spending 30 minutes of quiet, meditative time seemed to successfully lower my anxiety level. It also enabled me to reconnect with my inner self. During deep meditation, I would occasionally hear a soothing voice outside of my own reassuring me that all would be okay in the end. There is no way to know whose voice was calling out in the midst of meditation, nor does it really matter. My personal belief is that these messages were emanating from my soul, directly linked to the divine. The messages served their purpose and were healing, empowering.

Around that same time, I started having another recurrent dream. In the dream, I had the ability to perform physical activities free from concerns about my heart. I relived a part of my life that I'd known from my earliest days as a child but one that was now gone. Growing up, I'd always had a football, baseball, or basketball in my hands and I played competitive sports throughout high school and college. Lyme disease had taken that from me. My weekly basketball pickup games with other medicine residents seemed like another lifetime ago — but not in my dreams.

One night, I dreamed I had a strong desire to go out for a run. Running had always been my way to escape the emotional stresses of taking care of people with horrendous cancers prior to the Lyme disease. It had seen me through the rigors of having to "publish or perish" (the mantra of academics) and secure grants to continue my work. Running was a time when I could breathe fresh air rather than the stale air of a lab or chemotherapy treatment room. Pushing my physical limits had always been a way for me to confirm that I was capable of doing more than I thought I could do. In this dream, the will was there, but so was the hesitant fear that exercise might trigger an arrhythmia. I remember slowly beginning to walk and then breaking into a run as it became clear that nothing bad was going to happen to me. In my dream I ran like a child. I ran further and faster than I had run in ages. When I awoke, I felt invigorated and interpreted the dream as if my subconscious was telling me to go for it!

I also tried other forms of complementary healing techniques. A friend was getting her license in a form of energy healing called Reiki. The Reiki practitioner glides his or her hands slightly above the body while the individual is lying down. The idea is to mobilize energy from the practitioner to the patient, to improve the balance of energy in the patient and stimulate healing..

It may sound strange that we can benefit without the practitioner ever touching us. But it makes sense to me because our bodies are bundles of energy. Individual cells are constantly generating and consuming energy, with the molecule ATP (adenosine triphosphate) representing the body's energy currency. Cells generate ATP through complex enzymatic reactions, using broken-down particles of nutrients that we ingest like protein, carbohydrates, and fats. Many experts believe that chronic medical conditions signal an imbalance in the generation and utilization of ATP and other components of the energy-producing chain in cells. Since the heart is a muscle that consumes a tremendous amount of energy in a lifetime, I was willing to try anything to re-energize my heart. After all, the impulse that generates a normal heartbeat is a perfect example of electrical energy. My heart's electrical energy was clearly on the fritz, so I hoped a boost of energy might be exactly what was needed.

Denise accompanied me on my first visit to see my friend for Reiki treatment. Face-up on the table and enjoying the meditative music, I knew, if nothing else, that it was going to be a relaxing session. The atmosphere was so soothing that Denise had nearly fallen asleep after just a few minutes. Eyes lightly closed, I was completely relaxed as my friend worked her way up from my lower extremities, never touching me, just using her energy to rejuvenate mine.

When her hands eventually hovered above my heart, I suddenly let out a scream, waking my wife and nearly frightening my poor friend to death. At the instant the Reiki therapist had her hands over my chest, I had a vision. I went from being a doctor stricken with an ailment in my heart to being a Roman centurion on the field of battle, a bloody sword piercing my chest. I could not say for certain if I had awoken from a dream or if I was having an hallucination, but it was so real that I actually felt pain.

Nothing remotely like this had ever happened to me. In the vision, I was crumpled on the ground, crying out in pain and anguish (that was the shriek that had woken my wife) because I knew I was dying. I remember being distressed that my family was back in Rome, knowing they would never see me alive again. Then, and this is the strangest part of all, I saw myself lifting out of the body of that dead soldier lying still on the battlefield, floating above the scene of death and carnage on the plains of some ancient land. I felt an intense sense of freedom and overwhelming peace, and then it was over. The entire scene disappeared and as if hurling through a kaleidoscope, I was back lying on the table in my friend's home.

For several weeks afterwards, I saw that Roman centurion in my peripheral vision, and his presence somehow became a comforting sight. I empathized with him and wondered if his experience could somehow be associated with my heart condition. He was stabbed through the heart in ancient times; I was dealing with an ailing and broken heart. Were we somehow connected? I couldn't help but believe we were.

I mention this episode — at the risk of sounding peculiar or whacky — for one reason — it demonstrates how little we really know about our bodies and our minds. Nothing in the universe is as intricate and complex as the human body, and it deserves our utmost reverence. A marvel of creation, the body is comprised of trillions of individual cells, each functioning as a mini-universe unto itself. Thousands of biochemical reactions occur every second, each one precisely regulated. The slightest disruption of this perfectly orchestrated cellular milieu can bring disastrous consequences. It is a miracle and a testament to the resiliency of the human body and spirit that more of us don't randomly fall apart.

I believe there are many sources of healing energy that cannot be prescribed, surgically implanted, or analyzed by blood tests. We need to learn how to access that energy source to heal ourselves and help others. Each of us has the ability to do that. Tapping into that infinite energy source takes practice, dedication, and refinement of skills. Based on my own personal experience, there is much to learn from seeking out gifted individuals and alternative healers — especially when we act proactively and in a preventive mode before we get seriously ill.

Arriving at the realization that we know our body better than anyone else allows us to regain control over our life. In most cases, however, it is the physician who recommends therapy and makes the final decisions. Far too often, the patient passively visits a clinic or spends days anxiously awaiting test results. Just sitting in a waiting room, surrounded by others who are sick, is enough to engender a sense of futility.

The mere recognition that we are in control of our own bodies and our own destinies can be a powerful first step toward true healing.

In my quest to find spiritual and emotional healing, I soon learned that when we become more attuned to our body and spirit, unusual experiences like my first Reiki experience can become the norm. I recall giving a talk to a very large audience of cancer survivors. I was on the same program as Bernie Segal, the well-known author and surgeon who helped people all over the world through his emphasis on the importance of humor and health, as well as his lectures on the power of the mind-body connection.

This was the first lecture that I had given to a large audience since my heart condition had been diagnosed. Much to my dismay, as I sat in the auditorium waiting for my turn to speak, I felt the unwelcome sense of impending disaster again. As a myriad of thoughts raced through my head, my heart began to beat erratically. What if an arrhythmia strikes while I'm on stage? What if the defibrillator goes off, shocking me in front of all of these people? By the time I was introduced, I was in a state of panic. My heart felt as if it were jumping out of my chest. There was no way I would survive this one-hour talk.

When I reached the podium and looked into the faces of the audience, a sense of warmth enveloped me. It was as if a blanket of pure love descended upon my shoulders. Before I could utter a word, my heart rate slowed to a regular pace and the anxiety disappeared.

There was no rational, scientific explanation for going from an erratic heart beat and state of impending doom, to a sense of calm and tranquility. Several months later, I was asked to read a poem at the memorial service for my patient and good friend Miguel. Reminiscent of the funeral for my friend

Jon, I again experienced a sense of impending doom. Waiting to read the poem, my fear of an arrhythmia striking in the midst of that solemn occasion sent my heart rate once again into a state of chaos. I was convinced that something horrendous was about to happen. Instead, once I climbed the stairs to the pulpit and looked out over the crowd of mourners, I felt the same sense of peace, love, and warmth. I believe it was divine intervention. I don't claim to understand any of these episodes, but I do know they are real and comforting. Yes, scientists have unraveled the human genome, a marvelous accomplishment, but we still know very little about our own human spirit. What defines each of us is not our bodies, genes, or the diseases that eventually befall us. It is our soul. And what do we know about the soul? Most of us don't know much about it since we are too busy focusing on the material world, including obsessing over our bodies. For me, these episodes were simply reminders that Someone was looking out after me. I would be okay and I shouldn't define my life by a medical condition.

It was from this place of peace that I made a life-changing decision in the spring of 1998. It was an epiphany. If I continued to live my life as I had done up to that point — working night and day and devoting all of my energy to patients and their families to the neglect of my own emotional needs — I would surely die.

It was that plain and simple. I needed to take control of my life again. And, to do that, I would need to leave Miami in search of a job that wouldn't kill me.

Although I know not from where you came,
I feel a kinship with you.
You were once a proud soldier looking invincible.
But now,
Lying dying on a desolate battlefield alone,
With no one to hold you or shed tears.
I cry out in pain,
As the sword enters your chest, piercing your heart,
Your rhythm slows as blood drains from your body.
I see that which you see,
A blazing sun adorning the pure blue sky.
Oh God, please don't abandon me!
I am cold and so alone.
Who will be with me in my hour of need,
Other than the wolves tearing at my lifeless body?
I am not the strong soldier that I appear to be,
I am afraid.
Now I feel your soul rise above your body into the heavens,
As we gaze down upon your still form.
A sense of sudden freedom and joy,
Of liberation and reunion runs through our veins.
I am told to let go,
Encourage you to enter the light.
But I cannot part ways yet.
For you are me, and I was once you.

I love you,
You are not alone.
I was there to experience your death.
You are here now to help me through life.

"Old Soldier"

As I cry out in despair,
"Dear Lord, where have you gone,
Don't abandon me."
Where once your love filled my heart with a brilliant white light,
Now only hollowness remains.
I long to hear the still small voice from within,
But instead hear only silence, the vacuum of emptiness.
Where have you gone dear Lord?
Without your presence I am nothing.
You know my innermost thoughts and desires.
Do you actually feel the pain that I experience?

I know that You will grant us the miracle we so dearly pray for,
A child!
Twice within our grasp,
Twice unobtainable.
You now have our two angels in Your presence.
We rest assured knowing they are bathed in your light.
Comfort us dear Lord; let us feel your love.
Fill the void left in our hearts.
Sanctify us with the miracle of birth.

excerpt from "Faith"

24

Confronting my own mortality made me re-evaluate my priorities. That process, in and of itself, was healing.

I had always focused on my profession, perfecting a level of personal care with my patients that I felt was required. I realized I was spending so much time on my patients that I was neglecting the most important person in my life: myself. And my health suffered from it.

In the process of re-evaluation I realized I had never allowed myself time to grieve for the two pregnancies that we lost. Instead, I jumped right back into my work, shouldering the problems of my patients rather than confronting my own. Instead of releasing the emotional pain that had built up inside, I walled it off, figuring that it would disappear if I ignored it long enough or could exercise more.

Instead, it festered into an open sore. When I look back at the poems that I wrote during the three-year period immediately after our two miscarriages up until the diagnosis of Lyme disease in 1997, I can see the influence of my broken heart. Although I wouldn't — or couldn't — openly face the pain, it was obvious in my poetry. I was dying inside.

One aspect of choosing to live meant changing my job. As fate would have it, a job opportunity arose in the peaceful, bucolic university town where I had spent four years as an undergraduate. The job was with a large pharmaceutical company and would enable me to continue my research in cancer biology while pursuing my dream of developing new drugs that would improve life for millions of people with cancer. Most importantly, I would have more free time to spend with my family.

However, I initially balked when approached about the job because I was afraid to make a change. It would mean stepping out of my comfort zone. I had never worked in a company setting before; I had always been in an academic medical center. My greatest concern, however, was also a practical one. What would happen when my potential new employer found out about my medical condition and discovered that I had an implantable defibrillator? Would I be viewed as too great a risk to hire? To put it bluntly, I was afraid to leave my old job since I wasn't sure a new employer would want me once they discovered my medical baggage.

I had recently been turned down for supplemental life insurance through the group plan for faculty members at the University of Miami. This is an issue that millions of us face when going out into the work force with a pre-existing medical condition. At the age of 42, I was deemed an insurance risk. My chronic disease and internal pacemaker/defibrillator placed me at high risk for obtaining life or health insurance. I was frustrated to be locked into my job simply because I couldn't afford to jeopardize health care coverage for my family and me. Despite realizing deep down that it was time to leave patient care for the sake of my health, I was initially reluctant to take that leap.

By the time I reconsidered the job offer, it had already been filled. I was disappointed and confused about what I should do next. Call it karma or simply being lucky, but no sooner had I found out that the position was taken than I received a call that the job was available again. Apparently, the last applicant had changed his mind at the eleventh hour. That was all the push I needed. Without hesitation, I accepted the position.

At the end of the summer in 1998, we packed up our home with our baby girl and moved. I had gradually increased my exercise capacity to the point where I was once again working out on the Nordic Track for 30 minutes four or five times a week, interspersed with swimming laps. I was feeling pretty good, tired at times, but nothing out of the ordinary considering what had become my new "normal" since being diagnosed with Lyme disease. Life was good and Denise and I felt we had nothing to complain about. We had weathered the storm, we thought.

Once we settled in our new home in Chapel Hill, North Carolina, I made a routine appointment with a cardiologist. I felt fortunate because she was on staff at one of the top medical centers in the world. One of my first questions was related to the extent to which I could exercise. I told her about my progress and how good I felt. Before she would provide an answer to my inquiry, she wanted to evaluate my heart function. The last time I had my heart function tested was a year prior. We knew that the Lyme disease had damaged the electrical system; however, I had always been told the heart muscle itself was fine, as confirmed by my most recent test. I expected that my echocardiogram would reveal much of the same benign information.

I took the echocardiogram test. It lasted about 30 minutes.

The next day, I received a call from the cardiologist. I was a bit alarmed that she would call me at work because we'd only met the day before, but I assumed she was just establishing a rapport with me since I was a new patient with a rather unusual case. I was already exercising more than the average male my own age without a pacemaker/defibrillator. The defibrillator had not discharged one time since the incidents in the Newark and Miami airports. I fully expected the green light, releasing me to exercise to my heart's content.

I took her call in my new office.

"Are you sitting down?" she asked.

I knew immediately something was terribly wrong.

"Yes."

"According to the test," she said, "your heart is functioning at about ten percent of normal capacity for someone your age."

The doctor recommended that I see a heart transplant specialist right away. After I heard the word "transplant," my mind went blank. My heart function had deteriorated to the point where my life was in jeopardy.

One minute I had my entire life in front of me, and now I wasn't sure I would live to see the New Year. I was at a new job, in a new city, with our newborn daughter. I felt entirely alone at the moment.

Heart block I could live with; the pacemaker ensured that. Heart failure was something entirely different.

Somehow I managed to drive home. I walked into the kitchen and saw Denise holding six-week-old Celeste, fast asleep in her mother's arms. I could barely tell her the news between my muffled sobs. I saw the confusion and fear in Denise's eyes.

I recalled a lecture I had attended as a medical resident more than a decade earlier. A prominent lung cancer specialist had compared the five-year survival of patients with metastatic non-small-cell lung cancer (which we as medical residents assumed was one of the absolute worst diagnoses you could have) to that of patients with severe heart failure. The lecturer described in great detail how the patients with severe heart failure had a worse prognosis than the patients with lung cancer.

Remembering his words and looking at my wife and infant daughter, I became hysterical. I was convinced I would die for sure, and rather soon. I thought about how Denise must feel. Her husband comes home and announces he is going to need a heart transplant. She has a newborn at home in a new environment without family or friends. I couldn't imagine how she must have felt.

"Neil," she said, her voice quiet and reasoned, "let's just do whatever we need to do."

I looked at her incredulously. How could she be so calm?

She repeated, "Whatever we need to do, that's what we're going to do."

I took a deep breath and instinctively reached for Celeste to draw her tiny body close to my chest. I held our daughter the rest of the evening as she slept.

I tried to be like Denise. Strong, positive-thinking.

But, while holding my tiny daughter, all I could think about was everything we would miss together.

Two hearts beat as one.
Communicating without uttering an audible word.

Then on a fateful day,
One heart inexplicably falters.
Perhaps haunted by a sense of despair.
Succumbing to the destructive toll exacted by the heartache of repeated disappointment.
Regardless of cause, one heart desperately yearns for healing.
Crying out through unimaginable horrific acts.

Listen carefully,
For my heart does speak.
A soft utterance at first,
Gradually increasing to a feverish pitch.
Affirming its unwavering love and gratitude for its mate.
Commitment to uphold the bond that nature had always intended.
An eternity of seeking its soul mate from thousands of imposters.

You have been here for me.
I have been there for you.
We will always be one for each other.

excerpt from "Two Hearts"

25

The next day, I called my cardiologist and convinced her to schedule a heart biopsy. I wanted to know if active inflammation was the culprit damaging my heart. I was concerned that Lyme disease might still be active despite the aggressive course of antibiotics I had completed. An active infection could still be treated and, hopefully, improve my heart function.

I also began to immerse myself in heart failure literature. I wanted to be an educated, not a passive, consumer (advice I gave to my own patients). We don't think twice about gathering information before we buy a new car. Why should our own health be any different?

I began reading everything I could find about the latest research into the treatment of failing hearts. In the process, I came across a study showing that patients with failing hearts often had increased levels of antibodies directed to key receptors on the heart muscle (technically called anti-beta adrenergic receptor antibodies). Elevated levels of these antibodies were believed to contribute to deteriorating heart function. In Germany, physicians were doing clinical trials to reduce the levels of these harmful antibodies, often with marked improvement in heart function. Of course, I was willing to try anything. The problem was that the work was being done exclusively in Europe, not the United States.

I was now on my second heart biopsy, an uncommon occurrence for a man in his 40s. I watched the cardiac catheterization procedure on the monitor overhead as doctors once again snipped pieces of my heart muscle. With each came the expected runs of ventricular tachycardia. Despite reassurances from the cardiology team, the first several beats of ventricular tachycardia alarmed me. Traumatic memories of being shocked were still vivid in my mind.

The pathology report turned out to be relatively uninformative. Although there was evidence of heart muscle cell death, there was no trace of an active infection or antibodies attacking my heart.

• • •

I felt depressed. I couldn't identify a treatable cause for my dramatic loss of heart function. So, I once again listened to my gut instinct.

I was determined to move forward with a positive attitude rather than dwell on a number like ten percent heart function. After all, it wasn't as if I felt that bad. I was working and exercising.

I wanted another opinion. Brigham and Women's Hospital in Boston, one of the Harvard teaching hospitals, has an excellent reputation in cardiology, so I decided to schedule an appointment to be evaluated.

Before heading to Boston, I started increasing my dose of CoQ10 along with two prescription medications to help improve heart function. From a scientific perspective, the potential benefits of CoQ10 in folks with failing hearts made perfect sense. It is a key natural component of the energy-producing mitochondria — structures in the cells of our bodies vital for producing the energy that keeps cells functioning. Since the heart is a huge muscle that expends a tremendous amount of energy, and therefore relies heavily on energy produced by mitochondria, it made sense that a failing heart should require more energy. Moreover, research studies had shown that people with chronic illnesses like mine were at increased risk for being depleted of CoQ10 (which could not easily be corrected through diet). Despite the controversies in the medical literature as to whether it actually helped, it seemed there was little, if any, danger in taking it and several potential benefits.

In Boston, I underwent a battery of tests, including an exercise test where they hooked me up to a device that monitors oxygen consumption to determine how well my body extracted oxygen from the lungs and utilized it during exercise. Poor oxygen consumption can identify individuals with heart disease who are candidates for heart transplantation. To everyone's surprise, my oxygen consumption was in the normal range, although probably not where it had been when I was running marathons. Still, that was great news. In addition, a repeat echocardiogram showed an increase to thirty percent heart function. Although that was not normal, it was better than it had been three weeks earlier when I first heard the news of my deteriorating heart function. There was even more reason for optimism when the transplant specialist assured me that a transplant was definitely not in my immediate future, although he cautioned that it still might be required sometime in the future.

I came home with a renewed sense of vitality and longing to resume my journey of healing. I had a new challenge: improve my heart function.

The conventional teaching was that the heart muscle itself does not typically regenerate. Once it's dead that was it. But scientists were coming around to the notion that heart muscle could in fact regenerate.

Once again, I began to read everything I could get my hands on related to the regenerative capacity of the heart. For me, there was no better way to recondition my heart than through exercise, which I committed myself to do religiously almost every day of the week.

The assurance that a heart transplant was off the table reinforced that part of me that did not want to have my life defined by a number or statistic. In general, I felt pretty good, all things considered. And I did not want to incorporate more bad news and negativity into my subconscious.

It is uncanny how many cancer patients who are told they have six months to live end up dying right around the six-month mark. I remember talking about this observation with my Reiki therapist who had an interesting theory. When first told that they have a life-threatening illness, she said, people tend to go into a state of emotional shock, exposing their subconscious mind to the power of suggestion. Being told by a medical expert that you will likely live only a certain number of months is then incorporated into the subconscious mind. When that number of months has transpired, the mind subconsciously instructs the body that it is time to die, and so it does.

I've seen so many patients with metastatic cancer who appear to be doing okay when it all falls apart on cue, at a seemingly predetermined time. I've seen them one week and they're fine, then they are dead the next week at — you guessed it — six months.

I once told a patient who was heading into a bone marrow transplant where the quoted odds of success were less than five percent, "If it works for you, it's 100 percent successful." He was still alive 15 years later. I'm not advocating this approach for everyone, and I certainly believe that people should understand the nature of their disease, treatment options, and the risks associated with each treatment. It is simply to say that if you believe from the outset that the treatment won't work and that you are going to die in six months because that's what your doctor said, then there's a pretty good chance that you will be dead at six months or shortly thereafter.

Maybe it's best that patients not ask for the statistics on the first visit with an oncologist (or cardiologist, in my case). In my case, there were no credible statistics that I would have believed anyway, and even if there were, I would have likely rejected them outright. As I have been known to tell my patients, "Make your own statistics rather than becoming one."

• • •

The mind-body connection is very real and it is powerful.

During my medicine residency I cared for a gentleman in his early 80s. He was in pretty good health. It wasn't as if he had any imminently life-threatening medical conditions. He lived with one of his grown children's family. Just before Christmas the family brought him to the emergency room. After an examination, we quickly determined that he didn't need to be hospitalized. When we turned around to talk with his family about sending him home, they were nowhere to be found.

I reasoned that maybe the family was heading out of town for Christmas and couldn't bring him with them, so they figured we would take care of him until they returned. It was certainly out of the ordinary, not to mention cruel, but I was okay with it since he wasn't requiring much, if any, care. We could talk through better options when the family returned, I thought.

In the meantime, he seemed to enjoy the company of his fellow veterans at the VA Medical Center, sharing stories about his time in the military. As Christmas came and went, he started to count down the days until his family returned to take him home. This pleasant and likable man, who could have been my grandfather, became a favorite of the staff and offered his help around the unit.

New Year's Day passed, still no family. His mood started to change from the happy disposition when he first arrived to one of despondence. He began to withdraw. He then stopped eating and drinking, and within a few days this otherwise relatively healthy gentleman died.

I am sure that we listed the cause of death as cardiorespiratory arrest (his breathing and heart stopped), but I believe that he willed himself to die. If we can literally will ourselves to die, then surely we can will ourselves to live — at least beyond what the statistics indicate.

I was determined to live a quality life beyond what the experts thought was statistically expected. I had a clear choice: incorporate the concept of heart failure into every cell of my very being or accept the fact that I had a damaged heart but not allow my heart dysfunction to define me.

The medical profession does a disservice to patients when we pigeonhole them into statistics. Plenty of people have beaten the odds and gone on to become their own statistic.

That being said, I was cognizant of the reality of my medical condition and willingly accepted all I needed to do to survive. I had accepted the pacemaker/defibrillator and, of course, took whatever medicines I needed to take. But if that's all I did, I would have abdicated the true power of the mind-body connection.

A big part of harnessing that power meant not allowing my mind to buy into the statistics. Had I become consumed by the negativity related to my diagnosis, I might have died in six months.

I didn't give up hope. I let faith help me persevere.

Sure, there were plenty of medicines essential to my survival, tests I must have, and interventions that I may have to undergo. But I knew there was also a reservoir of strength within — and sometimes we might not even be aware of this strength.

I knew all too well that we can't rely on a doctor for everything. As good as doctors can be, if they don't try to motivate patients to access their own source of energy, they miss an important aspect of healing.

In my medical career, I have seen the difference between those who harness their inner strength versus those who don't. The people who abdicate their power to somebody else forget that healing is a collaborative effort. As a doctor, I can write prescriptions for my patients that help in the process, but they have to be fully invested in their own healing and believe in it.

• • •

I was also beginning to realize that there was a purpose for what was happening to me. We come into this life with something to learn, a task to accomplish. If we knew beforehand what the lesson was, what would life be like then? Everything would be scripted, and we would know the ending before we even started.

Instead, I believe we are born with a blank slate. There comes a time when we face a decision and whatever we choose to do next — how we react to a certain crisis — determines the course of the rest of our lives. I don't think everything that happens is necessarily preordained, but how we respond to events and challenges determines a large part of what our life may become. What had happened to me up to this point was the past, history. I couldn't change it. I could only look forward. Sure, at times I wondered what might have happened if doctors had figured out what was wrong with me the first time I had a skipped heartbeat. Perhaps I would not have gone through any of this.

But if doctors had "cured" me early on, I probably wouldn't have changed jobs. And if I hadn't changed jobs, I would have missed an opportunity that was waiting for me around the corner.

26

I accepted a job in pharmaceutical research with GlaxoSmithKline (GSK).

My background had always been in academic medicine, not in industry, so there was a steep learning curve. I couldn't do the same research that I had been conducting in the university setting, but I told the powers at GSK that I would like to at least have a laboratory.

I was fortunate to have had a great boss with an extraordinary vision for how he wanted to build translational research in a large company. In the late 1990s, most drugs were being developed in a traditional way. Researchers identified the highest dose a human could tolerate without dying, and then gave it to all-comers. The name of the game was to get the drug on the market as soon as possible.

Company executives didn't necessarily want to spend too much time learning a whole lot about the drug. That would slow down getting the drug on the market and delay profits. Fortunately, my boss had a different vision for discovering the science around the drugs that we were developing. He wanted to deliver the best therapies possible with the maximum benefit to individual patients.

I had been at the company just a short time when I was told that I would direct the lapatinib program — the company's flagship oncology drug at the time. I was nervous because there were several other people at the company who had much more experience in the oncology group than the new guy straight out of academics. I was still trying to learn industry lingo.

Lapatinib was designed to help women (and some men) who were dying of a very aggressive form of breast cancer that expressed high levels of a protein called HER2 (HER2+). Young women in the prime of their lives were more likely to have HER2+ breast cancers. Women were dying from this incredibly aggressive disease that was historically incurable with chemotherapy. The need was urgent and the disease was deadly.

The clock was ticking — not only for the patients who were dying but also for us to find a solution. I was on a self-imposed tight timeline. Being a patient myself, I knew just how desperate patients with life-threatening diseases are for some kind of hope and more effective therapies.

I poured my heart and soul into the development of drugs like lapatinib. The entire time I conducted my research, my heart was functioning at just a fraction of its full capacity. The work exacted tremendous energy from me, and I came home exhausted almost every night, only to go into work early the next day.

The research goal was to develop a pill targeting HER2+ breast cancers (and potentially other tumor types that overexpressed HER2) in contrast to Herceptin, which was given intravenously. I was fortunate to be working with a dedicated team of exceptional scientists, and we took this new drug into humans for the very first time.

Much to the surprise of everyone at GSK, we discovered that lapatinib seemed to be particularly effective in treating one of the deadliest forms of breast cancer: HER2+ inflammatory breast cancers (IBC). Despite the development of aggressive combinations of potent chemotherapy drugs, surgery, and radiation therapy, there had not been significant improvements made in the overall survival of women with IBC in 30 years. This research became a driving passion of mine, because women with IBC were the most desperate of the desperate patients. They were the breast cancer equivalent of my heart condition because time was running out for each of them in the same way it was for me. Each patient was living with a ticking time bomb inside.

I met with phenomenal IBC survivors like Ginny Mason, who heads the IBC Research Foundation, a leading advocacy group for the disease. I asked for her help in trying to develop lapatinib in women with HER2+ IBC. One of the problems was that it wasn't popular to do clinical trials in IBC. Some of the experts who were advising GSK said that it would be crazy for the company to listen to me, claiming it would take over a decade to conduct the first clinical trials of lapatinib specifically ear-marked for IBC patients. Why would you want to invest that much time and money in such a foolish endeavor? the advisors asked. But the evidence in my favor was too compelling, and no one could make me believe otherwise.

We'd already had an earlier breakthrough with one of the first HER2+ patient we treated with lapatinib. As it happens, she also turned out to be a woman with IBC.

I remember getting calls on a daily basis from one of the more supportive senior vice presidents asking me, "Did you treat the first patient? Was there a response?"

Everyone was waiting to hear if the drug would actually work. The day her treatment results were delivered to my computer, I opened up the pictures and saw the "before" photos that were taken of this woman's disease prior to treatment. It was spreading all over her chest and back. She looked like someone with third-degree burns. But in the short period of time that she had been taking the drug, the disease had almost completely disappeared. These latest photos revealed that the cancer had literally melted away.

I could hardly believe what I was seeing. I remember getting on the phone, forwarding the pictures to the senior vice president and saying, "We've got a drug."

My heart was pounding — and not in a bad way this time. I just sat back in my chair and whispered, "Wow. This is it." I think if we could have joined hands over the phone line somehow, this man and I would have jumped up and down, singing the Hallelujah Chorus!

That really was the "ah ha" moment. When I saw the dramatic effects of the drug on her cancer, I knew there was no way I was going to be deterred from conducting a study in IBC patients. I literally put my job on the line to do it.

The detractors had said it would take us 10 years to complete the trials. We completed the first part of the clinical study in about 10 months. That's even more incredible when you realize that the entire process of developing and researching the drug took eight years, receiving Food and Drug Administration (FDA) approval for the marketplace in 2007.

I remembered what my father told me, on more than one occasion.

"Neil, to succeed in research, you need to take the path less traveled and not just do what everyone else is doing…be a maverick."

That's exactly how my father conducted his work. He was a true out-of-the box thinker. At some level he paid the price going against the grain at times, which was not always the easiest course of action. Yet, he stuck to it. And, ultimately, I had to do what was necessary for these gravely ill people, even if the decisions that I made were potentially unpopular from a company standpoint or unpopular with other physicians. I may have worked for a pharmaceutical company, but my responsibility was, as it has always been, to do the right thing for people with cancer. My decisions about how the drug should be dosed or how it should be given sometimes went against the "experts" in the field. In my heart, however, I stood firm for the things that I believed were going to be best for patients, especially since I knew lapatinib like the back of my hand.

For example, the dose of cancer therapies given to patients has historically been based on the identification of a maximum tolerated dose (MTD), which is the dose you can give someone without essentially killing them. With a few exceptions, there is very little scientific rationale for giving MTD doses of cancer therapies to patients. As a consequence, patients have frequently suffered severe side effects, often fatal, without solid evidence the dose they were given was optimal.

Unfortunately, there is often a mindset among some people within the pharmaceutical industry (and academic medical centers) to avoid deviating from the status quo, even if the status quo is not correct. At GSK, I made it very clear that my approach would be different, developing so-called tumor-targeted therapies differently. Rather than an MTD, I pushed for the identi-

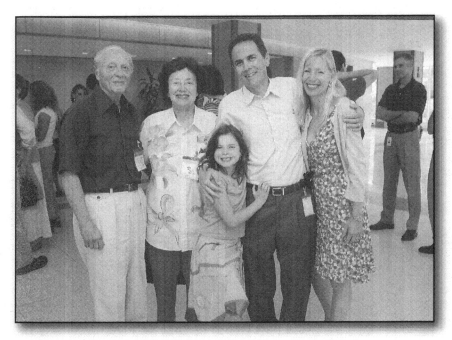

*(left to right): My father, mother, Celeste, me, and Denise
at a GSK party when I had 10 percent heart function*

fication of a safer, effective dose based on the identification of a biologically effective dose (BED) — that dose or dose range required to shut off the activity of the intended target(s) without increasing beyond that dose — a very different approach than the MTD. Identification of a BED would require obtaining sequential tumor biopsies prior to, and during, treatment as part of our early clinical trials. The naysayers — there were plenty — said it could not be done in patients with solid tumors. We did it. In addition, cancer drugs have in general been given to people without necessarily identifying those who are more likely to respond versus those who are not. If you give a drug at MTD to 100 patients, and only 10 respond, why subject the other 90 to toxic doses? I fought to develop targeted therapies in a targeted manner — identify those people more likely to respond, treat them, and then try to figure out why the others didn't respond and figure out how to help them. That seems reasonable. However, it wasn't well received among circles who wanted everyone to be treated. Identification of a subset more likely to respond would only reduce the market size of the drug.

I wasn't very popular among certain circles in the company. Thankfully, the people that I worked for in the research end of the company allowed me to be somewhat of a maverick.

But my commitment to these patients wasn't totally selfless. There was a part of me that wanted to believe there were other physicians and researchers who shared the same passion that I had, who were working tirelessly to develop new therapies for people like me with badly damaged hearts.

I prayed that a scientist somewhere was conducting research on heart disease and thinking, "I've got to get this new therapy out there so that people grasping for straws have hope." I wanted there to be someone with my best interest in mind over that of a company's, someone who, if he or she had a good treatment, was willing to stand up and fight for it even if others in the company wanted to make more money on an obesity pill because heart failure wasn't a big enough market. I hoped that there was someone who would stand up to the executives and even be willing to risk his or her job to do the right thing.

It is sobering to think that if I had not become sick, if I had not received the diagnosis of ten percent heart function, I wouldn't have been forced to change my life around. I wouldn't have saved a single woman's life with our work. I would probably still be at the University of Miami, eking out my research in a very small area.

Thank God my boss had the confidence in me that I could do something significant in research. Thank God I realized that I couldn't continue doing what I was doing in Miami and survive another ten years. I would have given away the remaining ten percent of my heart to my patients. With each grief-stricken family, my heart would have broken a bit more. I couldn't continue to be devastated every time somebody died. My heart had a limited number of breaks it could endure, and I'd reached my limit.

Waking up to the fact that there were not too many tomorrows remaining changed my life, and I like to think that it changed the number of tomorrows for the people who benefitted from the work that we did on this new drug treatment.

27

It turns out I could do a lot with only ten percent heart function.

Perhaps unwisely, I continued to push my attempts at living like every other man on my street. I would cut the lawn in 102-degree weather and forget to drink enough fluids. Even for the healthy among us, that's not a good idea. For somebody with an underlying disposition to arrhythmias, that's really not good because becoming dehydrated, which I did quite easily, could trigger arrythmias. Over time, I learned which activities would make me more prone to triggering skipped beats and potentially V-tach.

When I felt good, I tended to push myself to limits that I had no business testing. I was great at giving others advice about a healthy lifestyle, but I often didn't practice what I preached.

Staying up until three in the morning writing a grant would typically provoke flurries of skipped beats. I even tried to do things that I used to do when I was younger and healthy. Sometimes that got me in trouble. I desperately wanted to live a normal life. At times, it seemed outside my grasp.

Once while jumping in an inflatable castle with Celeste on a hot, humid North Carolina summer day, I suddenly heard the hum of my battery generating a charge. In front of my daughter and her friends, my defibrillator shocked me multiple times before my heart rate returned to normal. Imagine seeing your young daughter watching in horror as her father lay flat on the ground, gasping for breath, praying to survive the onslaught of electrocutions.

After that episode, I began experiencing anti-tachycardia pacing more frequently. I might have it several times a day for weeks at a time and then go for weeks without a single episode. I had learned to recognize the signs that the anti-tachycardia pacing was activated, dreading what was coming next should the arrhythmia continue. The burst of overdrive pacing could happen anywhere, anytime. If I felt it coming on when I was out walking the dog, I would find a place on the curb to sit down until those agonizing seconds passed. Sometimes it happened in meetings at work. I tried to casually wipe the sweat from my brow, breathe normally until it passed, and hope that no one noticed anything unusual.

On one occasion at work, I felt my heart racing out of control and, thinking I might pass out in front of my bewildered colleagues, I excused myself to go to the restroom. The bathroom was empty and I had enough time to grab the handicapped rail in the stall to steady myself until the moment passed. Feeling as if several hours had passed, although it was really just a few moments, I splashed some water on my face and returned to finish the meeting. These episodes were now regular events and just part of life as I knew it.

Overall, I was not in the obsessive, neurotic state I'd been in the year before, but still, I worried. For my wife, it was gut-wrenching to see me go through all of the mental torture of wondering when something was going to happen, as well as the physical pain when it happened. Living with someone with a heart condition or chronic disease not only impacted our family on an emotional level but also in the most mundane, practical ways. Planning a vacation or making plans to go anywhere away from home was scary because as much as I tried to downplay it, there was always the "What if…" factor to consider.

One time Denise planned a pool party with family and friends for one of Celeste's birthdays. I had just gotten out of the hospital for an episode where I had been shocked several times in a row and felt completely drained of energy. I could barely walk, fearful that each step might trigger a repeat episode of difficult-to-terminate V-tach. But Denise and I were committed to providing some sense of normalcy for our daughter.

She told me, "We've just got to do it. Even if all you can do is sit in the shade and watch."

And that's what I did. The photos of me sitting in a pool chair in the shade with a piece of uneaten birthday cake while everyone else was in the pool reminded me that this was the reality of our lives and we tried to make it work as best we could.

Despite my severely damaged heart, I was doing a pretty good job at everyday life. It's when my attempts at everyday life were punctuated by medical crises that things got hairy. Unfortunately, my crises tended to involve dramatic and unusual symptoms that seemed to have no explanation. Physicians have a term for patients like that—fascinomas. Trust me, you don't want to be the fascinoma. It's a made up term for patients with bizarre symptoms that don't fit any standard diagnosis. It's great if you are a physician taking care of a fascinoma because the cases tend to be so intriguing. If you're the fascinoma, however, it essentially translates to "good luck with that."

For example, after battling severe abdominal pain for weeks, a CT scan of my abdomen revealed a huge cyst the size of a grapefruit that looked as if it had partially ruptured. It was causing peritonitis — a dangerous inflammation in the lining of the abdominal cavity. At first, my doctors were concerned it might be a tumor.

In surgery, they made a startling discovery from a medical point of view. They removed a mesenteric cyst — one of the rarest abdominal growths in medicine. It was filled with a thick, dark fluid that had been leaking into the sterile abdominal cavity and causing the severe pain.

To me, it was just another example of "What the hell's going on in my body?" First I got Lyme disease. Then I got this dramatic cardiac complication that is not supposed to happen. And, finally, I have this rare mesenteric cyst. There isn't a documented direct link between Lyme disease and mesenteric cysts, but maybe mine was related. I was rapidly compiling a list of strange things that made me wonder what bizarre complication was next.

I did not have to wonder long.

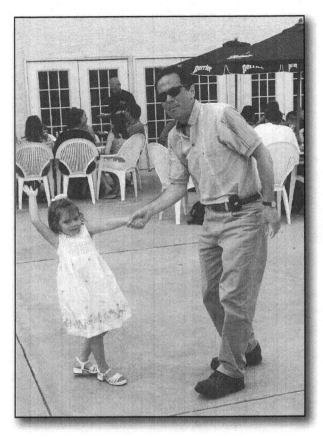

Dancing with Celeste

28

Every four years I had to get the battery changed in my pacemaker. When I initially received the device, I had read the pamphlet they gave me on what to look for if it malfunctions. One of the signs of an error or low battery was a synchronous set of ten beeps that would take place every 12 hours.

The pamphlet indicated that the beeps were likely a sign that something bad could happen, especially if the device was not sensing arrhythmia properly. *If you hear the beeping, get it checked out immediately.*

One morning I was in that twilight phase of sleep just before awakening when I heard what I could have sworn was a sports watch beeping. Denise thought it was our alarm clock. It stopped abruptly.

Later that evening as I was shaving to get ready to go on a date with Denise, I heard the beeps again. I realized the sound was coming from inside me, and I remembered the instructions about the low battery warning.

We called the doctor, but got a nurse because it was after hours. I described the beeping sound I heard, expecting her to confirm it was a low battery, but she proceeded to tell me it could have been anything other than the pacemaker beeping. Maybe it's my pager, she suggested. Maybe I didn't hear it properly. Maybe, she said in all seriousness, it was the telephone making the noise.

Why the staff screening phone calls often do not want to believe patients when they describe their symptoms is anyone's guess, but it happens to me, too, a physician scientist who reads all the pamphlets provided for devices and medicines.

The nurse eventually convinced me it was nothing, and Denise and I went to bed. Twelve hours after speaking with her on the phone, the series of beeps went off again.

I decided to see my doctor, who interrogated the pacemaker and immediately realized it was not functioning properly. For the past 24 hours, it had not been able to sense arrhythmias properly. Now they wanted to change the device.

When I wanted to run home and get some things to prepare to be hospitalized for the procedure, they wouldn't let me leave the room. Suddenly — ironically — I was on lockdown and it was no longer "all in my head." It was a dire situation that needed to be addressed immediately.

To me, this was such an obvious example of what happens if patients don't advocate for themselves. You can find yourself in big trouble.

So, what do we do if the medical professionals won't listen to us or refuse to believe what we're telling them? Be tenacious. Stick with your instincts.

I had known exactly what was wrong — it was described in the pamphlet, for God's sake. You don't get many definitive 10 synchronous beeping sounds in the middle of the night. Most of what I hear about what patients experience is nothing as concrete as 10 beeps every 12 hours. It's more of a vague headache or random pain that they can more easily be talked into dismissing. It isn't anything to worry about, they're told, so they ignore it. If that conclusion doesn't sit well, pursue it.

If your gut instincts are that this isn't right — I'm not supposed to be feeling like this, I'm not supposed to be losing weight like this, I'm not supposed to be beeping — keep pushing until someone listens to you.

If healthcare providers do not trust Denise and me — reasonably informed medical professionals — to describe a potential medical emergency, who are they believing?

• • •

Patients are up against a less human, less empathetic medical profession. As medicine becomes more technologically advanced and less personal with respect to patient/doctor interaction, being your own best advocate is going to be even more important.

It has been important in the past, but it's going to be vastly more so in the future because patients will be spending less and less time with a doctor, who will be spending more time at a workstation looking at a genomic analysis, or filling out electronic medical records, and precious little time looking at you, and listening to you.

In the future, doctors will simply look at a result from your human genome sequencing (essentially a map of every gene in your body) and that'll be "you." If you have a headache, there will be a little arrow on the computer screen pointing to a headache gene. And if a headache gene says you shouldn't have a headache because it's not red on the scan, then whether you have a headache or not, someone's going to tell you that you should not be having a headache.

Some people are saying you won't even need a doctor in the future. You will just punch in your symptoms on a computer screen or access an app on your smart phone. Your gene sequencing data would already be pre-programmed in and it will cross-match your symptoms, spitting out care instructions like a gas receipt.

I realize my opinion is not going to be popular with the in-generation of molecular medicine people. If people want a doctor who doesn't talk to them, then that's great — if that's the kind of care they really want. I just don't think most lay people will appreciate it once they understand what it entails. Personalized medicine is coming to America's doctors' offices, and it's not going to mean you're getting more personalized care.

Personalized medicine may in fact mean more automated, and less personal, care.

• • •

In 2004, it was officially time to replace my pacemaker battery again. However, this time doctors wanted to put in a biventricular pacemaker with an extra electrode wire that was supposed to help simulate a normal heartbeat by stimulating both lower ventricles to beat simultaneously. This new generation of pacemakers looked promising because studies had shown adding the extra kick was beneficial for some people with severely impaired heart function.

I prayed that this advanced pacemaker would improve my situation. It would make a tremendous difference in my life if it would help my heart function increase to just thirty percent rather than ten percent. I was upbeat and even excited about the potential, thinking maybe this was what I needed. I was holding out for that one missing piece that could catapult me to living fully again.

Unfortunately, the new pacemaker did not do what we hoped; my doctor was not able to position the extra wire in the optimal place to provide the added benefit. Although I now had the Mercedes Benz of pacemakers, it didn't do anything more than my old Honda Civic version. Maybe in the next four years when it was time for the next battery change, they could try again to reposition the wire.

I was disappointed, but I also had a new twist in my ongoing saga. I'd had echocardiograms at least once a year since 1998. In the early part of 2000, my annual tests revealed that my weakened heart was starting to expand like a balloon. For the first two years of my diagnosis of ten percent heart function, my heart was still a fairly normal size — just functioning very inefficiently. The human body is amazing, however, and it is able to compensate for diminished heart function. This is what allowed me to continue doing the activities I enjoyed, like going to work, exercising seven days a week, coaching my daughter's YMCA soccer teams, and mowing the yard. But as the years progressed, the size of my heart steadily grew and the muscle itself started to thin out, which resulted in even less efficient heart pump function. Imagine a garden hose full of water with a kink in the middle of it. As the part behind the kink expands to hold the water, the lining of the hose starts to get thinner. That's what was slowly happening to my heart.

Not only was my heart not pumping as efficiently as it should, it could no longer compensate as well because it was gradually losing muscle mass. I was destined to continue getting shocked periodically whenever the pacemaker/defibrillator sensed an arrhythmia.

In the summer of 2006, I was having a great time swimming with my daughter, Celeste (who was now eight years old), in our neighborhood pool. It was a warm summer day and the pool was filled with kids and parents. I suddenly sensed my heart racing. Within seconds, I heard the hum of the defibrillator charging and began to feel dizzy. I frantically swam to the side of the pool as quickly as I could, screaming out for Denise, who was talking with neighbors on the pool deck. She started running towards me with terror in her eyes.

Fortunately, another neighbor recognized something was terribly wrong and tried helping Denise pull me out, but it was too late. When the shock went off, Denise actually felt the jolt, since water is such an efficient conductor of electricity. How were they going to get me out if they keep getting shocked whenever they touch me? Meanwhile, Celeste was huddled nearby with a towel around her shoulders, silently watching everything take place. I started turning blue and by the time they finally pulled my body onto the deck, the defibrillator went off a second time. I rolled onto all fours, praying out loud to make it stop, when I got shocked a third time.

Boom, boom, boom! I was basically incoherent, but I remember thinking, This is it. I am going to die right here in front of my family, friends, and neighbors. By the time I was shocked the third time, my lips were purple. I was pale as a ghost and shaking from head to toe from the release of every molecule of adrenaline in my body. The sudden surge of electrical current throughout my body always left me with uncontrollable shakes and teeth chattering for 30 minutes to an hour afterwards.

It isn't as if life just returns to normal after getting shocked by a defibrillator. I would be physically drained and emotionally distraught since each defibrillation meant taking ten steps back. No matter how good I felt or what perfectly normal activity I was doing at the time, getting shocked was like someone smacking me in the face and saying, "What do you think you are doing? You've got a bad heart." It was a reality check — and I didn't like it.

Someone called 911 and the EMS arrived at the pool a few minutes later, along with the fire trucks. Our neighbors were getting used to this. Whether during the early evening, late at night, or in the early morning hours, they often heard the sound of sirens blaring louder and louder as they approached our neighborhood. I hated — and was guilt-ridden — that my daughter had to endure these events. Unfortunately, it wasn't restricted to the Spector household.

· · ·

Coaching Celeste's YMCA soccer teams throughout her elementary school years was priceless. It was a blessing to spend time with her and her close friends, teaching them a sport I loved and had played in my younger days. The last game of the 2008 fall season was in early November, the time of year when it is almost dark by six in the evening. I didn't even mind the chill in the night air because I was feeling good, running up and down the sideline, clipboard in hand, cheering on the girls. Suddenly I felt the pacemaker spring into action with overdrive pacing.

Oh, no — not here, I thought, looking down the sideline and trying to catch Denise's attention while I made my way to the ground.

I hit my knees, a wave of nausea and lightheadedness came over me, and I rolled over onto my back. Out of the corner of my eye, I saw Celeste looking at her dad sprawled on the ground as Denise and the other parents rushed over to help.

One girl on the team started crying, certain I was dying. Thankfully, the defibrillator didn't shock me, but the pacemaker issued several rounds of overdrive pacing one after the other and left me too weak to walk to the parking lot. One of the parents drove his truck onto the field so they could load me up and take us home. I was frustrated and upset, but too exhausted to think about how many more of my attempts at normalcy seemed to be falling by the wayside.

I had continued living a pretty normal life — and in some ways a more active one — than most people who have normal heart function. But the downhill slide had begun when my heart started to dilate. The heart can enlarge only so much before the thinned out muscle mass can no longer effi-

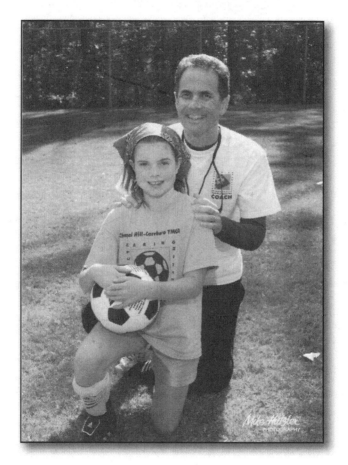

Coaching Celeste's soccer team

ciently pump blood through the body. My doctors knew that was the turning point, even if I wasn't ready to admit it. Although I had continued my rather strenuous exercise routine, I sensed that I was becoming even more fatigued. It took me longer to bounce back from workouts. Something very wrong was now happening inside my body. And for the first time, I had no idea how to redirect it.

Why just this morning I awoke to find an angel.
Although she lacked wings,
She was adorned with golden hair.
And when she spoke,
Her words resonated within my soul,
Assuring me that I was her charge,
To care and to comfort,
Sharing love and life for all eternity.

But God sent me his most precious angel.
The love of my life,
My wife.

excerpt from "My Angel"

29

Many people work their whole lives in the pharmaceutical industry and are never involved in a successful drug development program. Most drugs, even ones that look promising at the start, end up failing. By 2006, I had been fortunate enough to be involved in the successful development — and eventual FDA approval — of two drug therapies.

I now had the opportunity to take a research position at Duke University and assume a leadership role in the developmental therapeutics program at the Duke Cancer Institute.

I had worked with a lot of people at Duke in the laboratory and in the clinic over the eight years that I had been at GSK. I saw a tremendous opportunity in a university medical center setting like Duke to do exactly what I wanted to do, which was to continue to do research that would make an impact on patients' lives. Duke University is a tremendous academic institution, and the medical center is world class. Having a university associated with it brings access to a wealth of resources, including the chemistry department, the school of engineering, and one of the best biomedical engineering programs in the United States. This complemented my vision of taking great research and trying to benefit patients by translating the results to the clinic. Leaving GSK certainly wasn't as difficult as the decision to leave the University of Miami. I was able to continue my work in the laboratory, studying why drugs work for a certain period of time and then stop working, and discovering ways to make them more effective.

I was initially re-energized by the change in work environment. The research was going well and I enjoyed mentoring oncology fellows.

There were new challenges and stresses that I had not faced at GSK. Writing grants to support my research and my lab personnel, and cover my own salary, was very stressful and time-consuming, often requiring staring at a computer well into the early hours of the morning for days on end. By 2008, it had taken a toll on my energy. The winter of 2008 was a particularly difficult time.

It was also time to replace the battery in my pacemaker/defibrillator once again, which meant doctors could once more try to reposition that extra electrode in a more muscular part of my heart. What would have normally been a 45-minute procedure to change the battery turned out to be a long and painful task as they worked around significant scar tissue, trying to move the wire into a better position within my heart.

In the end, they were again unsuccessful. Nothing had changed in my circumstances, other than the fact that I had endured this painful procedure and had to take pain medicines for weeks afterwards because of incapacitating, shooting pains down the left side of my neck, shoulder, and arm. My chest now looked like a war zone with scars from multiple incisions over the years. The muscles in my chest, left shoulder, and back were severely atrophied, and I had several nerves that had been cut during the multiple battery replacements. All of this on top of a frozen shoulder that I had developed after the first pacemaker insertion. Simply put, I was a mess.

By early 2009, I labored to walk up hills that only the year before were not a problem. Paths that I had always taken at work now required several stops along the way to catch my breath. At first, I only stopped once and usually made a phone call as an excuse for why I couldn't walk uphill. A month later, I would need to stop twice. In the spring I had a terrible bout with the flu. The high fever exacted a toll on my body, triggering an increasing frequency of V-tach episodes, nearly all terminated by anti-tachycardia pacing. Due to third-degree heart block, my heart rate under the most intense workout was generally 100-110 beats per minute, so the threshold on my pacemaker/defibrillator to sense an abnormally fast rhythm had been set at 120. A threshold is a good thing, because it allows the heart rate to increase appropriately in response to exercise or other strenuous activities. Anything below 120 was not treated by the device. Anything above that was treated with either overdrive pacing or electrical shock.

During my bout with the flu, I experienced slow ventricular tachycardia at only 117 beats per minute — just slightly below the 120-beat threshold required to activate overdrive pacing. The slow V-tach had fooled my Rolls Royce device into thinking everything was okay. Realizing that the slow V-tach just under 120 could degenerate to a more deadly arrhythmia at any moment, Denise dialed 911 and off to the ER we went. The fix in the ER was rather straightforward. The doctors simply lowered the pacemaker's threshold to 115 — a relatively simple procedure using a small wand connected to an external computer to reprogram the pacemaker. When they waved the wand over the pacemaker and lowered the threshold, it immediately recognized the arrhythmia, went into overdrive pacing, and treated it without issue.

While I rejoiced in the minor victory of avoiding a shock by simply re-programming the device, I continued to deteriorate. Daily routines I had taken for granted for years were exhausting. Even walking up the stairs in our house from one floor to the next proved difficult. A parade of ambulances and emergency personnel came to our house on the outskirts of town at all hours, day and night. The cacophony of sirens could be heard in the distance growing louder as EMS and the fire department approached our neighborhood and then pulled into our driveway. It wasn't unusual during the late spring of 2009 for Celeste to wake up with a neighbor staying at our house because Denise and I would have had to leave for the hospital. We got to know all the EMS workers by their first names.

It was ridiculous.

I certainly wasn't ready to say that this was "the end," so I tried to approach the problem rationally. Maybe I was working too hard. Maybe I could modify something else and correct what seemed to be a pretty clear deterioration in my functional status. For the longest time, I believed there was a missing drug that had not yet been administered to me that would make all the difference. If such a miracle treatment existed, I felt the time was right to give it a try since I had taken a turn for the worse. I needed to last long enough until scientists perfected stem cell therapies to regenerate hearts.

There was an element of denial that I was experiencing the natural course of a fatal disease. I never resigned myself to the fact that, one, I could die from this; and two, I would actually need to have a heart transplant. They had told me in 1998 during my visit in Brigham and Women's Hospital that at some point I'd probably require a heart transplant, but I could not believe that point was rapidly approaching. Before this downturn, I had started thinking I could actually get by this way for the rest of my life.

Now, I knew better.

One early morning in mid-May 2009, Denise and I were awakened from deep sleep by a loud pop that seemed to have originated near my side of the bed. I had just rolled over, so I thought maybe I had knocked something off of the nightstand. The next day, Denise pointed out a small, wet spot over the pocket on the left side of my shirt. I didn't think much of it at the time.

A few days later, I got out of the shower and noticed a small opening in one of the many scars dotting the left side of my chest. Surgeons generally try not to cut along a previous incision because it tends to heal improperly and without the same strength as normal tissue. Over the years that I'd undergone multiple surgical procedures with my pacemaker, they had cut open the same scar repeatedly and then tried to close it with sutures. It had evidently not healed properly since my cardiologist had replaced the battery several months prior.

That opening was the "pop" Denise and I had heard. The doctors suggested in early June that I take antibiotics to see if it would miraculously heal spontaneously without having to do something drastic. I was feeling pretty debilitated at this point, although it's a funny thing because I had gone to the gym for a workout with my dad just the month before this incident. There were bursts of energy where I could do just about any activity, and then there were the more typical periods where I felt as if I could barely walk.

The doctors were concerned that the open wound could become infected and communicate bacteria from the skin directly into my heart via the pacemaker wires. That possibility had deadly implications. A few days before my daughter's birthday, I agreed to have a PICC line inserted in my arm so I could be at home while receiving an antibiotic intravenously over the next six weeks to prevent infection and hopefully heal the wound opening. The insertion of the PICC line was essentially an out-patient procedure. No big deal. When I got to the hospital late that afternoon, they couldn't do the procedure, so they suggested I spend the night in the hospital, put the PICC line in first thing in the morning, and then be discharged home.

Denise was with Celeste on a school trip at the North Carolina Zoo an hour and a half away. I called Denise on her cellphone, and explained what was going on. It was pouring rain and I could hardly hear her above the noise of the sheets of water slapping against the nearby window.

She asked me if I thought she should leave so she could be with me.

"Don't worry," I told her. "Have fun today. Stay dry."

"Bye, Daddy," I heard Celeste say in the background.

I planned to be home in the late morning in plenty of time to celebrate at Celeste's birthday dinner the next day.

• • •

I eventually drifted off to sleep, which was difficult for me to do in the hospital. I awoke to the sound of people hovering over me, talking in what sounded like an alarmed tone. It was 3:30 in the morning and several doctors and nurses were standing around my bed.

"What's going on?" I asked.

Everyone was looking at the heart monitor near my bed. I looked up at the monitor and saw that I had a normal blood pressure.

That's good, I told myself.

I could tell I was thinking clearly. That's good, too, I rationalized. So why the concerned look on the faces around my bed?

To my surprise, I was once again in slow ventricular tachycardia at a rate just below the threshold where the pacemaker/defibrillator senses an abnormally fast rhythm. I calmly explained to the medical team (residents, and a cardiology fellow) exactly what they needed to do to lower the threshold, thinking I would make their job easier. After all, this had happened once before and was easily treated by lowering the threshold. However, instead of listening to me, the patient (and what's more, a physician like them), they decided to inject me with a potent anti-arrhythmia medication. Nine out of ten times that would have been a safe and correct choice, just not in my case. Remember, I am the fascinoma.

Within seconds of receiving the medication, I knew something was terribly wrong. It started as a sickly, warm sensation — a familiar signal that I was in impending danger.

I remember saying, "Oh my God, I think I'm dying."

"Get him to the ICU," someone yelled. That's the last thing I remember.

When I finally came to and opened my eyes nearly seven hours later, the first thing I felt was relief that I had made it. My wife was sitting vigil at my bedside, holding my hand. I remember thinking, what is she doing here? I told her to enjoy the zoo.

She began filling me in on all that had happened, starting with a call she'd received from one of the residents in the middle of the night saying that I was in slow V-tach. She had told them to reprogram the device, just as I had. Ten minutes later, she got another, more urgent call.

"You need to come to the hospital as soon as possible," the voice on the other line said. "We can't tell you anything more on the phone. Hurry." That's code for your loved one is dying and you had better get here ASAP.

When she arrived at the hospital, I was unconscious with my feet up in the air, the bed completely tilted because I had essentially no blood pressure. Denise explained that they'd had to do CPR since they couldn't feel a pulse. I noticed that I had bitten my tongue and had abrasions on my head, apparently from a seizure that I had due to the lack of blood flow to my brain. Worse yet, my arm was severely swollen. When I checked in to the hospital the previous afternoon, I had only been given a flimsy IV for fluids since no one anticipated a life-threatening emergency would occur. It was not appropriate for the powerful medications I would end up needing at 3:30 am to increase my non-existent blood pressure. In the rush, they tried to force the drug dopamine through the tiny IV line, despite the potential for it to leak and cause serious tissue damage. As a result, the medicine had seeped out from the vein into my skin and caused massive swelling in my forearm.

There is only so much swelling your arm can accommodate before the tissue starts to die in a condition called compartment syndrome. The treatment for that condition requires filleting open the patient's arm to relieve the pressure and cutting away dead tissue to reduce the risk of infection. People can lose limbs due to severe compartment syndrome. Now that I had survived my brush with death, we anxiously awaited the plastic surgeon to determine what needed to be done with my arm.

I've read books about the idea that we have three check-out moments in life — near-death experiences where you can decide to leave if it's your time. This was definitely a check-out moment for me. If my soul had been ready to exit, this would have been the moment. I had no measurable blood pressure for several hours. That could have been a check-out moment for the healthiest of individuals, let alone someone with 10 percent heart function. People with underlying cardiac dysfunction generally don't make it through something like that.

After Denise told me everything that had transpired over the past seven hours, all I could think was that I must not be ready to die yet. It was like a revelation. They can say what they want, I thought, but this heart is pretty damn strong to get me through all of this. My blood pressure eventually returned to normal and my arm, though still swollen, would not require further treatment.

They discharged me later that afternoon. Just as I'd originally planned, I was sitting at my daughter's favorite restaurant the next night having dinner for her birthday.

I went from near death to trying to figure out what I wanted to order from the menu at Elmo's Diner. I should have been at my own funeral service, but instead I was eating a veggie burger with my family.

Time was running out for me. I knew it. Denise knew it. After this overnight experience in the hospital in June, I began having 15 to 20 episodes of ventricular tachycardia a day.

Any one of them could kill me.

Here I am Dear Lord,
Amidst the commotion of the moment,
Doctors and nurses moving in a chaotic dance,
Fear and desperation etched in their facial expression,
Fixated on the constant bellowing of alarms monitoring my essential functions.
Their fear has now become part of my existence,
Even as I try to make light of the situation.
My energy is draining from the constant pounding of an arrhythmia.
Strange how such a fast rate could lead to such a feeble pulse.
I sense that my brain is starting to shut down, starved of vital oxygen.
My heart cries out for help,
But I am helpless, unable to stop the onslaught.

My beautiful wife, radiant with angelic glow even at such an ungodly hour,
Tries hard to comfort me, "everything will be alright."
I want to believe, but thoughts race through my mind,
Did I tell Celeste how much I love her?
Can I leave this existence without saying goodbye to so many that I love?
Is this my time or has there been some cosmic mistake?

Oh God, where are you in my greatest time of need?

Can you not hear my prayers through the din of the moment?

Are you speaking to me?

Am I unable to comprehend your answers as my sensorium fades?

Do I take my last breath with your name forever engraved on my lips?

Every instinct tells me to fight and pray for deliverance from this nightmare.

And then it happened.

"Do you feel different?"

For a moment I wonder about the origin of this seemingly strange question,

Coming from my wife, who is gazing up at the monitor.

Yes, I do feel different.

Lights are suddenly brighter, voices clearer, and my mind is sharp again.

My heart no longer racing, unexplainably the arrhythmia terminating
spontaneously.

The nurse, whose expression was one of despair only minutes earlier,

Is now praising You Dear Lord.

No plausible medical explanation can account for this dramatic turn of
events.

Only prayers answered and Divine intervention.

Thank you God for being there, in the midst of human chaos,

Holding me high above Zion,

And delivering me from harm's way.

Thank you for the Gift of Miracles.

excerpt from "The Gift of Miracles"

30

No one outside of Denise and my doctors knew how close I was to a life and death situation every day. For all intents and purposes, I looked like anyone else in reasonably good health, except that I had to go through a separate line at the airport for a pat down because of the pacemaker/defibrillator.

But I could no longer hide the fact that my health was deteriorating. I look back on June and early July 2009 as six weeks of hell. First, I still had the hole in my skin overlying the pacemaker and the concern about a serious infection remained. In lieu of a PICC line, my doctor prescribed an oral antibiotic for six weeks. I knew the antibiotic was critically important. Within a few days of starting the medication, however, I began to vomit every time I ate something. For someone who had regurgitated maybe twice in his life, it was demoralizing not to be able to eat without getting violently ill. It was a living nightmare.

Second, the episode in the hospital with dangerously low blood pressure for seven hours had taken a toll on my poor heart. Experiencing episodes of V-tach day and night without an obvious provocation was exhausting. I wasn't doing strenuous activities at that time, since I was too weak from not being able to keep food down. The arrhythmia would come on even while I was lying down resting. Fortunately, anti-tachycardia overdrive pacing successfully treated each episode. Had I been shocked 15-20 times a day, I wouldn't be here.

My doctors finally put me on a powerful anti-arrhythmia medication (the same medicine that they had injected into me earlier when I thought I was going to die), but this time I took it in pill form. I was admitted to the hospital for the first dose because I didn't trust taking the medication at home. God forbid I would have a repeat severe reaction. Thankfully, I tolerated the drug without problems, and within a short period of time it suppressed the arrhythmias. The nausea, however, continued.

I was admitted to UNC Memorial Hospital in late June to try and control the constant vomiting. The first night, I asked for a sleeping pill and anti-nausea medication. Within an hour of taking the medication, I started hallucinating, probably as a result of the combination of the sleeping pill, nausea medicine, and low blood flow to my brain. I was in the hospital room by myself trying to listen to my iPod, but I was having trouble concentrating. Staring at the earbuds in my hands, I could not remember how to put them in my ears. Was I beginning to lose my mind, too?

I later became convinced that there was somebody in my room, crouching over in the corner like a lion ready to spring. I got out of the bed and called out to the nurses in the hallway to help me. I even called my wife in the middle of the night, telling her that somebody was trying to kill me.

She tried to calm me down, assuring me there wasn't anyone in my room and encouraging me to just listen to my music and relax. But I wasn't thinking clearly enough to know how to work the iPod. As the night went on, I was terrified by visions of people all around, closing in on me. There was a part of me that objectively knew it wasn't really happening, but the hallucinations seemed so real.

· · ·

With the dramatic change in my health, Denise and I felt it would finally be a good idea to meet the head of the Duke heart transplant program. I still wasn't at the point where I had accepted transplantation as the next step. Dr. Joseph Rogers was a wonderful man with a great bedside manner, the type of physician you would want taking care of you in a difficult situation.

When I walked in his office for our appointment, he asked incredulously, "You walked all the way here from the parking deck?"

I nodded. That day was actually a relatively good one for me.

After I gave him a brief medical history, he couldn't believe what all I had been through. After he examined me, he explained that while he could put me on the transplant list, he didn't think I was in a dire situation. Several criteria determine the order of the transplant wait list, and I wasn't at the point where I would go to the top of the list. If he put me on the transplant list based on his examination that day, I would likely be waiting quite a while. I was relieved and left thinking I'd just received some pretty good news. Maybe I was going to beat this after all.

Several days after our visit, however, I experienced an irreversible turn of events. The nausea had wiped me out, and my energy level was non-existent. I began having a new and almost indescribable symptom. Some people suffer from the agony of restless leg syndrome (RLS), where they have an irresistible urge to move their legs or other parts of the body in an attempt to relieve a painful sensation. RLS sufferers often can't find a comfortable position to lie down or sit. It ultimately interferes with their sleep, which compounds the misery.

I started experiencing a head-to-toe sensation of not being able to get comfortable in any position. A dull, aching, and often throbbing sensation coursed throughout my body. It was relentless and quickly driving me crazy. There were nights where all I could do was pace around the house. I'd sit in a chair, but I couldn't stay there for long because every muscle in my body started to ache. I'd then try to lie down with pillows propping me up, but I couldn't do that either. I tried to watch TV to distract my attention from the torment of the pain, but that didn't work. Forget meditation or listening to soothing music when you are already miserable and the only thing you want to do is escape from your body. In a nightly ritual, I roamed my house while everyone else was asleep, wide awake and feeling tortured. In retrospect, the restless body syndrome was probably related to my deteriorating heart function and the poor perfusion and oxygenation of my muscles.

For the first time in this entire 16-year ordeal, I started to feel as if there was no way out. I was falling headfirst into a ravenous black hole that was sucking all the life out of me. Why couldn't I just die? I did not want my family to see me suffer a gruesome, prolonged death like this. Death is a blessing when someone passes unexpectedly in the night. It's not a blessing when you realize that it's going to be excruciating for you to experience and equally excruciating emotionally for your loved ones who have to watch you die.

Far above my dread of cardiac arrhythmia, the greatest fear that I'd always had was of being in physical pain all the time. I'm not talking about not being able to walk or get about anymore, which would have been bad enough. I'm talking about being miserable every moment, every second of my life. Not being able to eat anything, not being able to think clearly.

There are many examples of inspirational people who do incredible things given their physical limitations and still enjoy their lives. However, I felt like I had no escape from constant misery, and I was now at a place of utter desperation. Never in my wildest imagination could I have envisioned reaching this point.

I considered taking my own life.

Denise and I had never discussed assisted suicide but I could understand the way somebody with Lou Gehrig's disease might feel. Like me, they might be totally repulsed by a glimpse into what life would be like in the near future. Who wouldn't want to take a more peaceful way out?

We don't allow our pets to undergo excruciating deaths. We put them to sleep in a humane, peaceful way so they won't suffer. No patient has ever asked me to help him or her in an assisted suicide, but I've been in many intensive care units watching families grieve in situations when the overwhelming odds are that that their loved one is not going to make it.

In all the times that I was being shocked by my defibrillator, lips turning blue, trembling uncontrollably, unable to put two coherent words together, I never once thought, *That's it. I can't live through this anymore. I have to end it all.*

However, there was an evening in June 2009 when I saw my wife sitting at the kitchen table and a plan began to formulate in my mind. She could administer an overdose of morphine and let me die peacefully. I just wanted to be out of my misery. I hadn't been able to eat in a month without getting sick. I hadn't slept in a few weeks because of this horrendous restless body syndrome. It was the perfect storm for reaching the breaking point.

I went to Denise that night, held her hand, and told her how much I loved her. But I needed her to do me a favor.

"I can't go on living like this," I said, choosing my words carefully.

I'll never forget the expressionless look on her face. She had no words. I don't think she believed I was serious. I had never uttered anything remotely like that in our entire marriage. Plus, she had already resigned herself to the fact that I was going to get a heart transplant. In her mind, my condition wasn't terminal. We still had options. I would soon be on the transplant list and the worst would be over.

I, on the other hand, wasn't thinking "transplant." I was thinking, This is my life now. It was not going to get better, despite all of the positive faith and determination to overcome my adversities that I'd had for so many years.

Suddenly, the reality of my situation overwhelmed me. Every ounce of strength that I had was not sufficient to overcome the desire to end it all. If there had been a gun in the house that night, I would have put it to my head and pulled the trigger.

It still hurts to revisit that night in my memory, but it makes me realize that given the right circumstance — or maybe the wrong circumstance, depending on how you look at it — anyone is capable of coming to that conclusion.

We know people who have committed suicide, or even people who have attempted it, and we sometimes call it an act of weakness or mental illness. However, someone's marital distress, financial duress, or medical illness can lead anyone to that point. I'm convinced of that now more than ever.

I just thank God the opportunity wasn't available for me to act on it.

The impulse was so strong for that one instant: I needed to die.

You have given me a renewed purpose to live.
Each moment is precious and unique,
Never to be experienced again.
With each passing day,
You grow and change,
A new gesture,
Curiosity at the world around you.

As you grow,
I want nothing more than to be by your side.
Helping you pursue your dreams.
For dreams do come true, my little Celeste.
As your mother and I have discovered.

A father's dream has come true.
I no longer need to look forward to rocking you in my dreams.
For you are here in my arms.
I love you little Celeste!

excerpt from "Celeste"

31

As suddenly as the urge to commit suicide had come upon me, the impulse passed. I returned to the hope that the discovery of a cure was still out there. Someone would come out of a lab, shaking a vial, and say, "I've got it! This is going to work."

I might die, I told myself, but it would not be at my own hand.

• • •

Now that my arrhythmias were better controlled, my cardiologist wanted to readdress the issue of the hole in my skin overlying the pacemaker. Several weeks of antibiotics had only made me sick as a dog without healing the open wound.

Although I had no visible signs of infection, my doctors were still concerned that the hole exposed the pacemaker to bacteria on the skin. The pacemaker was 12 years old and some of the wires were now firmly embedded into my heart tissue. Pulling on these wires would certainly rupture my heart. The procedure they planned would put a sheath around the wires and use a laser-like device in an attempt to free them from the heart tissue. Again, rupturing my heart was a very real possibility.

My cardiologist was very experienced at inserting pacemakers, but he had very little experience removing pacemaker wires that had been implanted for a long time. He was very honest in telling me up front that he wasn't sure how the operation was going to turn out because it carried such high risk. He considered the procedure medically necessary, but I wasn't so sure. We set the date for the procedure after the Fourth of July holiday.

For the first time facing a surgery, I was scared. I knew that I might die during this procedure. We had sent Celeste to Florida with my wife's cousin and her family to be away from the craziness that had descended upon our lives. Rather than keep her at home to witness the sadness that had become our daily routine, we sent her to play on the beach.

Knowing that I might die during the procedure, I sat at the kitchen table and performed one of the most difficult tasks of my life. I wrote a letter to my eleven-year-old daughter.

I wrote about how much I loved her and how long I had prayed that God would deliver a miracle child to us when that didn't seem possible. I wrote about how proud I was seeing her grow and take on challenges without being afraid to fail. I wrote about the little things — coaching her soccer teams, telling her bedtime stories, gazing at the stars. These were the best moments of my life and ones that I would miss the most.

I wrote about all the events in her life that I would not be around to share. Her graduation. Helping her learn to drive, just as my father had done with me. Being at home on her first date and giving her boyfriend a hard time, like all fathers are obliged to do. Being there for her when her heart broke for the first time. Taking pictures at her high school prom. Walking her down the aisle at her wedding. Experiencing the birth of a grandchild. Marveling at the young woman she had become and taking great pride in the accomplishments and contribution to society that she would surely experience.

I sealed the letter, several handwritten pages in length, and gave it to my wife, who promised to give it to Celeste should I not survive.

• • •

The only reason my heart was even continuing to beat at this point was because of the pacemaker. If they took that out, even temporarily, what was going to sustain my life? I would have a heart rate of 30 beats per minute, which wasn't going to do me any good. And removing the pacemaker meant removing the defibrillator device — the electrical shock system that had already saved my life many times. What would happen if I had V-tach without a 911 system in my chest?

The doctors decided to install a temporary pacemaker so that I would at least have a heart rate of 60. There was even talk about a hi-tech vest, which sounded more like medieval torture than medical innovation. The vest's wire linked me with an external defibrillator and generator poised to deliver a powerful shock if I had any arrhythmias. My prospects did not sound great, especially if I needed to sit in a hospital bed for several weeks with nothing more than a vest and a single pacemaker wire keeping me alive.

It was not a pretty thought, but it seemed like the only option because the consequences of having an infection spread to my heart would have been deadly. We decided to go ahead with the procedure.

What was supposed to be the easy part — putting in the temporary pacing wire — proved to be difficult. But it was vital before the surgeons could attempt to remove the old pacemaker. After hours of labor, the temporary wire was in place.

The anesthesia alone could have been life threatening for me. Anytime a patient with 10 percent heart function and a history of ventricular arrhythmias goes under anesthesia the risk of death is high.

The day after inserting the temporary pacing wire, they wheeled me down the hall to surgery. I gave my wife the thumbs up sign, silently communicating that it would all be okay and we would soon be back on the road to something, though I couldn't say what. However, within minutes of giving me general anesthesia, my blood pressure dropped to a dangerously low level, and the doctors aborted the procedure.

I woke up in recovery, assuming that the surgery had been successful. I turned to my wife and gave her a weak smile, but her face told a different story. She reached out to touch my hand just as the cardiologist walked in, who also looked as if he were about to burst into tears. He explained that they had to stop before they could even get started because my blood pressure had bottomed out.

"I'm sorry, but we just can't go on," he said.

I didn't want to think I was out of options, but I didn't know what else we could do at that point. The cardiologist didn't offer any ideas either.

I had a pacemaker that should come out, but couldn't. My blood pressure couldn't tolerate surgery. And, my heart was failing.

Just when I thought it couldn't get worse, it did.

32

I was in the shower when I noticed that I had started developing a belly, as if I were getting a beer gut from downing six-packs. It was the day after being discharged from the hospital following the failed attempt to remove the pacemaker. Initially, I didn't know what to think about this unattractive development, but over the next day or two, my abdomen started to get bigger.

I realized my heart had taken a final hit. I was in full-blown heart failure and accumulating fluid.

I had always prided myself on maintaining my physical fitness despite having 10-15 percent heart function. Prior to 2009, I never took a diuretic and never had significant swelling in my ankles — which was in some sense a miracle because edema (fluid accumulation leading to swelling) is a symptom of declining heart function. Now, however, my slim frame was swelling all over. I looked as if I were six months pregnant. Next the fluid started building up in my lungs, forcing me to sleep sitting upright in order to breathe.

My body was shutting down. My kidney function was deteriorating, and my liver function was being affected because my heart wasn't pumping sufficient blood. I also wasn't getting enough blood to my brain, but in the midst of my jumbled thoughts, one thing became evident.

This is it, I told myself. This is what it's like to know you are dying. Make no mistake about it, I was dying.

• • •

I was readmitted to the hospital to start diuretic therapy to try and get the excess fluid out of my body. It was a tricky process since my blood pressure was only 80/50, and the diuretic therapy could very well lower it even more. I am not sure how successful the hospitalization was since I still had significant total body swelling. Perhaps suspecting that I would soon be readmitted and wanting me to have a day or so at home, my doctors discharged me from the hospital with an oral diuretic pill I could take at home.

That didn't last long. At home, the swelling rapidly progressed. My legs were like balloons and my abdomen was so swollen that I was unable to fit into my regular pants. Denise had to buy me stretch pants that would accommodate my swollen torso. My feet no longer fit into my shoes, even sneakers with the laces untied. The sight of my body at this point reinforced the fact that I had entered a new phase in my struggle. Lyme disease had not only ravaged the electrical system in my heart and crippled my heart's pump function, but it had now destroyed any resemblance of the man I was before I got sick.

As I looked like a six-months-pregnant woman, my wife responded by doing something that may have saved my sanity. Unable to wear anything but the largest stretch pants and consciously avoiding looking at myself in the mirror, I felt anything but sexually attractive. However, one night she set the stage for what turned out to be an intimate romantic evening of pure bliss. For that period of time, I felt whole again. She knew that I was dying and would likely die without a heart transplant, even before the doctors made that point explicitly clear. Perhaps she thought this might be our last passionate moment together. At that moment, we lived as if there were no tomorrow, only the present. And the present that evening was a gift. It was a brief reprieve from the nightmare that had become our reality.

The next day, I ended up back in the hospital.

One of the dieticians brought me a smoothie one day — a nice, small gesture that meant a lot to me. In the midst of all that was going on, there were still bright lights along the path that reminded me how good life could be, although they seemed like they were few and far between.

My sister-in-law and her women's prayer group in Delaware were also praying faithfully for me, along with other small groups of people who had heard about my story. They would pray earnestly for my life every Wednesday night. I had another friend in N.J., an old high school classmate, who prayed for me every night at 9:00 pm. She told me, "I want you to pray because I'm praying." And I would. In my hospital room, I prayed as I'd never prayed in my life. I would listen to encouraging songs that my sister-in-law's group had given me, just living off the faith of others at that point.

Death, I had learned, was not necessarily a continuous, downward spiral. I continued to experience periods of miraculous recovery, however temporary they were. One day I was on death's doorstep at the hospital, and then the next day I'd be out walking around the halls telling my doctors, "Hey, I feel pretty good." My ashen appearance would suddenly improve and my team of doctors would look surprised and say, What's with this guy?

On days when I thought I was better, I'd convince myself that they just needed to give me that magic prescription they'd been holding back to fix this thing and I'd be back to work, doing what I was doing before.

But now I had a catheter inserted to collect urine because my kidneys were not functioning properly, as they were not getting enough blood flow. My body seemed to be shutting down. Something was meant to happen, but it wasn't my death.

I still wasn't ready to accept the fact that I needed a transplant, even though the cardiology team and medical transplant experts were now stopping by nearly every day to encourage me to think about a transplant.

"Have you thought about transplant?" Members of the transplant cardiology team at UNC would come into my room to say. "You know, it's not a bad thing. Just think about it."

Of course I had thought about it — but for whatever reason, I wasn't ready to give up on my heart.

33

I didn't want to abandon my heart. This was the heart I'd had for 53 years, the heart that experienced my first kiss and first time falling in love. It was with me when I saw my daughter for the first time, and it was there as I sat with patients, watching them take their last breaths.

I knew my memories would still be there, but I wondered if the emotional connection to them would be altered if they removed my heart. Of course, I would remember holding my daughter for the first time, but would it be the same? Or would it all change? It was hard to conceive of losing a part of my experiences all at once. Imagining losing your heart and getting another one; this is what I thought about.

I had always thought of my heart as the two of us against the world. My heart and me — that was it. We could do this. It was more than an organ in my body. The seat of the soul, my heart, was part of my personality. I wasn't ready to concede the fact that I was going to lose it forever. It had weathered the storm with only 10 percent function and sustained two potentially fatal episodes with barely detectable blood pressure, events that would have likely been too much for even the healthiest heart to handle. As weak as it was, my heart had gotten me to this point. It stuck with me. It was determined to see me through, and I somehow felt as if I couldn't leave it now.

As strange as it seems, I wasn't thinking about how much I needed the transplant to survive. I was focused on what life was going to be like for me from a spiritual standpoint.

Over the years since discovering it was damaged, I had developed a spiritual connection to my heart. I talked to it regularly and visualized it being encased in healing light to open up whatever chakras were blocked — whatever bad karma was happening in the heart. I concentrated on treating my heart with loving-kindness and prayed for the chance to let me get it through this.

I would silently say to my heart, the doctor said you shouldn't have made it through, but you did. So, stick with me, I'll get you through this.

I knew things were bad — really bad. But I wasn't making plans to say goodbye. Outside of the one time that I asked Denise to help put me out of my misery, I never felt as if I were on my deathbed awaiting last rites. Despite the fact that I looked like I was about to deliver twins and my organs were shutting down, I just knew it wasn't my time to go.

This was not it.

On Friday afternoon, July 17th, the doctors arranged to put in a Swan-Ganz catheter, which is a catheter inserted into your neck that is then threaded into your heart. The success of this procedure is tied to the heart's ability to help thread the wire where it needs to go. The contraction of each heartbeat moves the thin wire along from atrium to ventricle so doctors can measure the volume and pressure in the heart. This would tell them which medications and how much they could safely give me to remove the fluid accumulating in my body, without dropping my already precariously low blood pressure even further.

I had performed this very procedure myself at least two dozen times during my medicine residency training, so I didn't think anything of it other than as a routine procedure for someone in my situation. I couldn't breathe well lying flat because of the fluid in my lungs. However, I had to lay still on the cold slab of a procedure table as they carefully tried to thread the catheter into my heart. It took longer than what seemed necessary to me, and I began struggling to breathe. My skin color was ashen gray from the lack of blood flow and the antiarrhythmic medicine I was taking. The cardiologist was very experienced (he was the director of the cardiac cathaterization lab at UNC), but he was having a difficult time getting my barely beating heart to move the wire. An hour-and-a-half had passed since the procedure began when he finally gave up. He compared it to trying to sail a sailboat on a completely windless day. He held up a fist and made a slight quiver to show how poorly my heart was contracting.

They returned me to my room and I told Denise and my parents what had happened. That's when the head of transplant surgery walked in and introduced himself.

"Do you want me to sugarcoat this or just tell it like it is?" He was an imposing figure, standing beside my hospital bed.

"You'll be dead by Monday unless you have a heart transplant. Otherwise, you're not going to see Monday. You need to make a decision. You have 72 hours."

I was suddenly transported back to the times when I'd experienced the ethereal, peaceful warmth during some of the most intense episodes of arrhythmia over the past 16 years. As the surgeon continued talking about my options, I once again felt a soft blanket of pure love wrapped around me. I was the most content I had ever been in my life, as if God's angels were cradling me in their arms and protecting me from fear.

"You need to give up control, and let us take over," the surgeon continued. "You're trying to control the situation, thinking there's a mystery drug out there we're not giving you. You've been trying to take care of yourself, trying to be your own doctor. Stop doing that. You're going to fail unless you let us help you make these decisions."

When he said that, the light clicked on. I found myself in one of those defining moments where I knew what I needed to do. I needed to let go and let God take over.

I don't necessarily think that's what the surgeon had in mind when he mentioned giving up control, but it's exactly what I heard.

I thought to myself, he's right. I've done all I can do. The rest is up to a Higher Power. There was nothing more left for me to do. Whatever was meant to be, it was up to God to take care of it at that point.

This was on a Friday in July of 2009. I was 53 years old.

• • •

It's difficult for others to understand this strange feeling I had when I was told I was going to die if I didn't get a heart transplant, but I was in a state of overwhelming serenity. I was completely relaxed, absolutely calm. They took me back down to the cardiac cath lab to insert an aortic balloon pump, a large catheter inserted into the artery in my groin and threaded up into the aorta, the main artery carrying blood from the heart to the body. It would now take the pressure off my failing heart. The balloon pump immediately stabilized my rapidly decompensating heart function so I could be transported safely to Duke University to be enrolled on their heart transplant list.

I remember the balloon pump making a soft swooshing sound with each heartbeat and thinking it was the most beautiful rhythm I'd ever heard. It was all somehow meant to be now. It's happening, I told myself. The grand scheme is coming to fruition. If a transplant is what was supposed to happen, then this is what the plan is. If this is what the plan is, I'm giving up my control to God.

Every burden, every ounce of extra weight on my shoulders, was now somehow gone. I wasn't merely saying or thinking, I have faith — I had given it all over to a Higher Power. I had surrendered.

And I never thought that I was not going to make it through whatever I was about to endure. Not for a minute.

I did not know exactly what was going to happen to me in the next 72 hours, but I felt certain that I would not die that weekend.

34

For anyone who has faced a life-threatening disease, it's best to seek out the very best care. For me, that meant moving seven miles down the road to Duke University Medical Center, where they have one of the largest heart transplant centers in the United States. I was in the ICU at UNC Memorial Hospital Friday evening waiting for the life flight crew to transport me early Saturday morning to Duke. I was trying to lay as still as possible so I wouldn't disturb the catheter in my groin, still listening to the reassuring cadence of the balloon pump. As the hours went by, I came to love that sweet sound. It was keeping me alive.

I am a firm believer in the power of prayer. A friend of mine surprised me with a quick visit, just to tell us that everyone was praying for us. Then another family came in and recited Psalm 91 by heart. My friends gently draped a prayer shawl over me as they recited the psalm, a wonderful gift for someone facing death. Two young men who went to church with my administrative assistant also came to my bedside and anointed my head with healing oil. God's angels in Heaven and on earth were always by my side.

Later, the nurses gently gave me a bath and let me sleep most of the night. I ended up having the best night's sleep that I'd had in weeks, falling asleep to the swooshing sound, a lullaby to my ears.

• • •

In the early morning, the Duke life flight team arrived, jovially claiming to be "rescuing me" from the University of North Carolina, their bitter rival in the sports arena. As they wheeled me outside, I saw the earth was wet with rain from the night before, and I breathed in a lungful of fresh, dewy air. I'd been living in a hospital room off and on for weeks now, and the unexpected cool July morning was refreshing. One of the UNC nurses that my wife and I had become very close to gave me a hug and assured Denise that God was going to take care of me. As they loaded me onto the ambulance, I noticed the cardiology fellow who had provided me such compassionate care over the last week of my UNC admission. He stepped forward out of the morning shadows of the loading dock and handed off the CD of images of my cardiac studies. I noticed tears welling up in his eyes, as if he were saying farewell to a dear friend — a powerful gesture coming from a doctor who knew my case all too well. Then one of the Duke life flight nurses placed a small brown teddy bear in my arms, a gift to give to my daughter, and a gesture that touched my heart.

After a short ride in the oversized ambulance that was more like a miniature hospital on wheels, I arrived at Duke University Hospital. I had been walking these same halls only weeks before in my lab coat, passing a menagerie of patients on the health-disease spectrum. Now, I was the one people were looking at, vaguely intrigued by the machine keeping rhythm at the foot of my gurney.

I was feeling energized by the ride over to Duke, but an ominous sense was brewing inside my wife that things just weren't right for some reason. Denise had a dream — a disturbing dream the night before. In her dream, we entered the world-class cardiac care unit at Duke only to find it was a dingy, overly crowded and confining place that smelled like a county hospital. As I was wheeled into the ICU, she realized her dream was based on reality.

It was obvious that I needed a transplant very soon, but everything had happened so quickly that they hadn't even determined if I was a good candidate for transplant. The first thing the Duke transplant team wanted to do was a right heart catheterization to make sure my lungs had not been damaged by the pressure from heart failure. I'd already experienced fluid build-up, but they wanted to confirm that I had not yet developed pulmonary hypertension, a permanent condition where the pressure in the blood vessels of the lungs is dangerously high.

Failing this first test would have put an end to the heart transplant right there. Doctors don't want to put a new heart into somebody with bad lungs that will eventually destroy the new heart. The test might have revealed I needed a heart-lung transplant, which would have brought a whole different set of challenges.

Unfortunately, they had to attempt another Swan-Ganz catheter as part of the procedure (which had already been an excruciating exercise in failure at UNC). To my surprise, a fellow was assigned to do my procedure. A first-year fellow in any other profession would be called an apprentice, someone who is essentially starting at ground zero and trying to learn everything he or she can. Along with him was a resident, someone even more junior in rank and experience. I'd just come from a top university hospital where the head of the cardiac catheterization lab had tried in vain under the most optimal of conditions, and now these two were going to attempt the same procedure at my bedside. I was hardly in a position to argue as I was basically immobilized, unable to move my upper body past 30 degrees because of the aortic balloon pump.

Denise and I pleaded with them not to try it, explaining what a colossal failure it had been just the day before. Nevertheless, they insisted they could do it and asked my wife to leave the room. Threading a very large catheter through my groin and up into my nearly exhausted heart was painful, distressing and bloody. Forty-five minutes later, they left as anticipated, without success.

Unbeknownst to me, the ICU room was spattered with my own blood from their efforts, soaking into the sheets and covering the floor. I watched helplessly as Denise cleaned it up herself, silently taking her anger out on the linoleum floor. Was this another bad omen at the start of my 72-hour interval between life and death?

Early on Sunday morning, doctors moved me to the cath lab so they could attempt to insert the Swan-Ganz catheter under better conditions. This time, the procedure worked and the results showed that my lungs were fine. I so appreciated the warmth and levity the cath lab team of nurses and assistants brought to the situation — joking with me about a Tar Heel from Chapel Hill "having the nerve" to call them into work on a Sunday morning.

"We go light on the sedation for Tar Heels," they teased good-naturedly about lowering my pain meds.

They knew I was on the verge of dying. They knew my circumstances were dire. But instead of acting as if they were preparing for my funeral, they helped me anticipate a good outcome. We shared an unexpected laugh together in an area of the country where sports rivalry finds its way into everyday life, even the cardiac cath lab.

Potential obstacle number two was convincing the transplant team that I did not have an ongoing infection in the pacemaker pocket. I still did not think that was the case, but there would be no transplant until any infection was treated and resolved. If the team thought the small hole on my skin was an active infection, I might stay in the ICU on a balloon pump for weeks or even months, receiving intravenous antibiotic therapy. Since I would be immobilized with the aortic balloon pump in place, all of my muscles would atrophy. They might have to retrain me how to walk (assuming I lived long enough to get a transplant), since my time was limited even with the balloon pump. Fortunately, after a consult with an infectious disease expert, I won the argument, proving I did not have an infection and could proceed with the transplant.

The transplant surgeon came in soon afterwards to talk about officially putting me on the transplant list. It was noon on Sunday now, and the UNC's surgeon's words repeated themselves in my ears: "You'll be dead by Monday . . ." *Would the clock run out before I could get a heart?*

"You need to decide if you are willing to receive a high-risk heart," he said.

Denise and I looked at each other with blank expressions. What was a high-risk heart? I wasn't sure. Someone with an infectious disease? An elderly individual? The possibilities flashed across my mind, but I couldn't imagine they would transplant a heart with any physical defects.

The surgeon went on to explain that a high-risk heart has nothing to do with the physical nature of the heart. It is a heart from someone who was a prisoner, had a history of being a pedophile, was a drug addict, or a sex offender.

"Some people have a hard time with this," he offered, choosing his words carefully. "Some people don't. I will tell you that these high-risk donors tend to be younger people who otherwise have healthy hearts."

There wasn't time to linger over the issue because if a heart became available from that high-risk pool, then the transplant team needed to know whether I was amenable to accepting it or not.

The decision wasn't an easy one even for someone like me whose heart was barely pumping blood. Taking any heart seemed like the rational choice. But the prospect of receiving the seat of someone else's dark soul reminded me of the offbeat movies I'd seen where the soul of the criminal is transferred into somebody else with disastrous results. Does accepting a heart from a pedophile come with experiences, whether I'm conscious of them or not? Is there something in every fiber of every heart that remembers the behavior of its original owner? I didn't know.

I knew they would test a drug addict's heart for HIV, hepatitis and the like, but what about the viruses that we don't yet know about that are communicated through intravenous drug injection? Maybe three years from now there would be a new virus that drug abusers get — and I would have a drug abuser's heart inside me. What then? In the end, we couldn't make a decision right then as to whether or not we would accept a high-risk heart. And, thankfully, we never had to.

My prospects for receiving the first available heart from outside of the high-risk pool were good because I was at the top of the transplant list. The reason I was there had nothing to do with privilege, since I was a faculty member at Duke. Being kept alive by the aortic balloon pump and powerful intravenous cardiac medications put me at the very highest risk of dying. I was in need of a transplant as soon as possible.

One of the other factors involved in deciding whether an available heart is appropriate for patients on the waiting list is the compatibility of the recipient and the donor's blood types (A, B, O, or AB). In many cases, the blood types are not compatible and the recipient has to wait for the right match.

Luckily, I had AB blood type, which is the universal recipient blood type. That meant I could accept any heart, from any donor, with any blood type. AB blood type is found in less than five percent of the population. For once, I was thankful to have another oddball statistic assigned to me. Of all the weird, textbook-defying things that had happened throughout my illness, having an unusual blood type proved fortuitous. Another advantage was that I am of average height and weight. If a potential recipient is 6'5", he or she would need a heart from a similar-sized individual and vice versa for someone of shorter stature. Everything was working in my favor for once, and I felt good about my options even though it was now Sunday evening and the clock was ticking.

Denise stayed with me for as long as she could before I insisted she go home to rest. I was officially on the transplant list, and it was now just a matter of time.

At 10:30 pm, the phone rang beside my bed. It was the transplant coordinator on the other line.

"Neil, are you ready?" she asked.

"Ready for what?"

"We've got a heart for you."

35

I called Denise on her cell phone and told her we had a heart. Of course, she started freaking out . . . literally, freaking out. The transplant coordinator called our home phone, so we were all talking rapid fire with both phones, asking questions and getting more information. When we hung up, Denise attempted to call me back but accidentally called our neighbor across the street instead.

"Oh my God, oh my God," was all she could say to my confused neighbor who had woken out of a deep sleep and assumed something terrible had happened to me. When Denise was finally able to get out the words, our neighbor ran over to our house to share in the good news.

I wasn't alone when I got word about the donor heart. Two friends, Simone and her son Josh, had driven from Washington D.C. that evening just to keep me company.

After a while, I put on my headphones, laid my head back, and listened to what I consider to be my saving grace song, *Healing Rain*, by Michael W. Smith. My sister-in-law and her prayer group had given me a CD with spiritual songs including *Healing Rain*. Denise and I had listened to it throughout the past few weeks, drinking in its encouragement that the healing rain was finally on its way to fill my dry heart.

There is typically a four-hour window between when the transplant team harvests the donor heart (removes the heart from the donor) and when they have to insert the organ in the recipient. It was approaching midnight now, and I assumed the transplant team was flying somewhere in a jet, although I didn't know where they were going. Once they arrived in the operating room

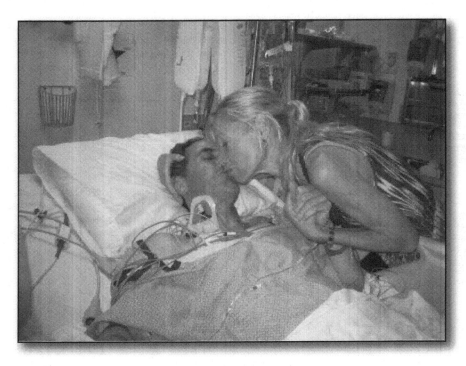

Several hours before transplant surgery

of the donor, they would have to make sure the heart was suitable for transplantation. If everything looked good, they would then pack the organ on a special mix of ice and chemicals before flying back to Duke, hopefully arriving about 2:00 am Monday morning.

I knew nothing about the donor other than the person was not in a high-risk category. In fact, the first words out of my mouth to the transplant coordinator when she called were, "Is it a high-risk heart?"

To be honest, if she had said, "This is a high-risk heart from a pedophile," I don't know what my answer would have been, but I was relieved to hear that it was not high-risk.

Denise soon joined Simone and Josh in my room, along with some other friends who came by when they heard the news. I was now counting the hours. Two hours went by. They still had to prep me for surgery, but nothing was happening. I tried to wait patiently, but at 3:00 am I started to panic that something was wrong. For the first time since I got on the transplant rollercoaster that weekend, I was nervous. The ICU tried to call the transplant team at the donor's hospital but could not reach them. I was now concerned to the point that I started thinking maybe the jet had crashed. All these dire scenarios were going through my mind, and I began telling Denise and my friends that maybe this had all been a cruel hoax because the heart must not be viable. I turned 180 degrees from being calm to thinking that this wasn't meant to be. It was torture.

This went on until 3:30 am. Then 4:30 am. No change. No news.

I was fervently listening for the sound of the helicopter blades outside my window because my room was located near the landing pad on the roof of the hospital. All I heard was the droning of the air conditioning. Sometime around 4:45 am, the nurses came into my room and said the words I had been so anxious to hear.

"We're taking you into surgery."

There wasn't much time to transition from despair to being wheeled away for my operation, but I was instantly back on track mentally, my balloon pump lulling me into a peaceful rest once more. I don't know what that last minute deviation was all about. Maybe it was a final test of faith, I'm not sure. Denise was holding my hand as I made the journey toward the OR. Patients can't enter the OR wearing any jewelry, so I slipped my wedding ring off my left hand and placed it in her palm.

"I'll see you in a few hours," I told her.

I was calm and resolute with a smile at the corner of my lips.

It would be a long wait before we would see each other again. And a new life was waiting for me in the OR.

When I arrived in the OR, one of the anesthesiologists introduced everyone in the room. One by one, they pulled down their blue masks and waved. They were cheery and eager for five o'clock in the morning. The anesthesiologist was wonderful. I remember him telling me that they would take great care of me, as he injected medications into my veins and put an oxygen mask over my face. That was the last thing I remember thinking before I was out. Denise later told me that she walked over to the window after I left her and saw it was raining. Healing rain had come to this old town, just as the song promised.

• • •

Denise, her sister, and our friends spent the next 12 hours in the waiting room. My father came later that morning and waited for the end of my surgery. Periodically, someone would come out of the OR to give them an update at certain milestones of the procedure, including a neighbor (an anesthesiologist at Duke not involved in my surgery) who also happened to be in the OR suite that day and peeked in on me to tell my family I was doing okay.

At the end of the operation, they put me in a recovery room only to usher me right back to surgery to stop some bleeding. The removal of the pacemaker and deeply imbedded wires had caused unexpected bleeding. Once they stopped the bleeding, I returned once again to recovery.

I later learned that my anesthesiologist talked to Denise after the procedure.

"If I had to have a heart transplant, that's the heart I would want," he told her.

He went on to explain how they often have to electrically stimulate the transplanted heart multiple times to get it beating again when they put it in the recipient's chest. However, all they had to do to mine was tickle it and it was raring to go.

Then, he told Denise another story from the OR.

Like two hearts passing in the night, he said my old heart was literally on its last beat when they removed it from my chest. It had hung in there, quietly pumping out a final few drops of blood, surrendering to the surgeon's hands only when it was certain it was no longer needed.

When Denise told me the story, I had the image of one tired heart being taken from the OR and the other coming in, eager for a new turn at life. For me, the exchange of energy between these two life forces was like the passing of a baton. One had been taking care of me for 53 years, and now it was the other's turn. One heart had made sure I got safely to this point. Now, another would need to take me home the rest of the way.

The medical director of the heart transplantation program at Duke also visited Denise in the waiting room when he heard what had happened during my surgery. He was surprised to learn of my operation, since this was the same man I'd spoken to only a month earlier when I didn't qualify to be at the top of the list.

"I'm just going to say this," he said to Denise, drawing a deep breath. "I've been doing this a long time and what's happened here today is nothing short of divine intervention."

In his mind, it was all a miracle.

Here's a guy who is steeped in scientific training at one of the top elite medical centers in the world. He could have come out of the surgical suite, looked at Denise and said, "Thank God for your husband's genes. You know, they really got him through this." But he didn't say that.

He could have said to my small band of loved ones in the waiting room, "Thank God for the surgical technology that got him through this." But he didn't say that either. He firmly believed that what happened was a true miracle.

My experience was reaffirmation of the fact that there is power in prayer, there is power in belief, and there is power in having faith. I think people are searching for something beyond the wondrous medical technology we have because they want to believe that we're more than just double strands of DNA. Why I believe in God and have faith and why I believe in prayer has nothing to do with DNA. It's more than just some gene that says I'm wired to believe that way. My friends and family don't recall the incredible technological advances at work in the hospital that day. They remember a physician at a major academic institution that prides itself on conducting top-notch research saying this transformative, life-saving event was divinely orchestrated.

It was tough on Denise to see me, post-operation, on a ventilator, heavily sedated in the ICU Monday night. Dozens of tubes, IV drips and monitoring wires were scary enough. Plus, she could not talk with me or hear my voice. When she saw that I was resting comfortably, the nurses sent her home for the night.

"Go home, get some rest," they told her. "The work begins tomorrow."

36

Coming out of the anesthesia a day later, I heard someone speaking to me, but I couldn't open my eyes.

"Squeeze my hand," she said. "That's it. Squeeze my hand, Neil."

I told myself that I had to squeeze this person's hand and let her know I was in here somewhere. It seemed this disembodied voice was coming from far away in a dark hall, but I didn't know how to respond.

"Take a deep breath now," the voice directed me next. I did and felt some pressure as they removed the breathing tube from my throat.

I took another series of deep breaths, my eyes still unable to focus.

Suddenly I was back.

I'm here, I remember thinking, as I looked around the room.

I then felt the strangest sensation inside my chest.

"Something's wrong here," I whispered to the nurse, my throat scratchy and raw from being intubated.

I pointed to my chest.

"There's nothing wrong, Dr. Spector. It's just your heartbeat," explained the nurse.

For the next 30 minutes, I insisted that it was beating too fast, too strong. It just didn't feel right at all. This thing inside me was pumping away in a super physiologic function. I should have been happy, but I was scared.

She calmly showed me that I had normal heart function. It had been over 12 years since I last experienced a normal heart rhythm without a pacemaker. I had forgotten what the beat of a healthy heart not regulated by electrodes felt like. I went from ten percent pre-transplant to completely normal heart function in one surgical procedure. In fact, all the indicators were that I was above and beyond the normal range. But for me, "normal" was disconcerting. For so long, an electrical pacemaker had initiated my heartbeat.

Now, I had a perfectly normal heart that was not only beating on its own but also pounding out of my chest. The intrinsic difference between a heartbeat and a pacemaker rhythm was startling.

"Oh my God, feel this thing," I said to the nurse, wanting to put her hand on my chest.

"It's like a natural heartbeat again," I said.

She smiled and nodded.

I was giddy. I had a strong, muscular heart ferociously beating within my chest, as opposed to the weak, thin, dilated muscle I had become accustomed to having.

I started laughing. I was exhilarated.

"Oh my God, this is unbelievable! Look at me!"

My color had gone from ashen gray to the rosy, pink flesh of a fully functioning human again. That was the first thing most people noticed when they saw me after the transplant. Friends confessed that they didn't know how bad my situation really was because they were accustomed to the ashen gray complexion I had before the transplant. Now, I looked like a newborn baby, cheeks flush with color.

It was still very early in the morning and Denise had not come back to the hospital yet. Next, a physical therapist came by and asked, "Do you want to get out of bed? Let's do some walking." I felt more than ready to test out my new heart.

The therapist helped me gather a skyline of IV lines and poles and tubes draining fluid from my chest so I could ease out of bed and walk with the assistance of a walker. My first few steps on the cold linoleum floor were triumphant. I had energy. I was not short of breath. I was feeling good and I was alive. After a few laps around the half-circle of desks inside the ICU, the physical therapist was ready to discharge me from his care.

"You're fine," he told me, a big smile on his face as I insisted on doing one more lap. "I'll just see you later."

He waved, shaking his head, as I embarked on my next lap solo. When Denise came, I was sitting upright in a chair next to the bed, grinning from ear to ear.

"I just walked around the ICU," I said proudly.

She could hardly believe it, since the last time she saw me I was unconscious on a ventilator. I have to admit that some of my elation was likely due to the high doses of steroids I'd been given to prevent rejection of the new heart. Steroids make anyone feel like Alexander the Great, ready to conquer the world. Between that and having a heart giving an olympic performance, doctors were soon ready to transfer me out of the surgical ICU into a step-down unit on the floor.

This was a momentous occasion because my daughter had not been allowed to see me in the ICU. We were finally able to see each other for the first time since she had left for Florida over a week earlier. Having her arms around my neck was a priceless experience for me, but I'm sure it was also probably incredibly frightening for her. I was alive, but to see the plethora of tubes coming out of every orifice other than my mouth and nose would be overwhelming for any eleven-year-old.

I started walking the halls several times a day. I knew exactly how many laps equaled one mile. The first day, I walked two or three miles. My daily pattern became walking one mile after breakfast. Then after lunch I'd clock another mile, followed by one more mile after dinner.

The nurses were amazed, albeit a little concerned. One said, "You know, you've got to take it easy. It's not like you just had your tonsils taken out. You just had a heart transplant, for Pete's sake."

I wasn't going to waste a single opportunity to start exercising my new heart. Everything had happened so fast the first week after my transplant that I didn't have time to think much about the consequences of my good fortune. In the first few days of my recovery, it began to sink in that my miracle was also another family's tragedy. The initial exhilaration of having this beautiful beating heart and hearing everyone tell me how blessed I was morphed rather quickly into somber thoughts about what it must have been like on the other side of the equation. My family was making laps with me, celebrating, while somebody else out there in the world was burying a family member.

That truth was difficult to deal with. How do you justify your life, knowing someone else had to die so you could live? Don't get me wrong. Going from being told on a Friday you are going to die on Monday to suddenly walking three miles in the hospital is thrilling. Aside from Denise, I never shared with anyone else my mixed emotions, because I didn't want to spoil their celebratory mood. I was walking, talking, eating, and smiling. People were hugging me and sending balloons to my room. In quieter moments, however, I could not help but think, *Why am I the one here?*

I also thought about all the other people on transplant lists who were not so lucky. Somehow I was here, while their families were still waiting on pins and needles for the phone to ring. Someone's mother, daughter, brother, or best friend was on the same nationwide heart transplant list I had been on — with the same hopes — but they wouldn't make it because they would go into cardiac arrest 12 hours or five minutes before their surgeries. Without a doubt, the majority of me was happy to be alive, but still a part of me focused on the greater reality.

For a long time after my surgery, I continued to struggle with experiencing these two opposite emotions at the same time. A friend finally explained to me that it was not as if I killed the person who was my donor.

"That person died and now their family has the opportunity to create something good in the midst of their grief," she explained.

She was right. It's not as if I were somehow responsible for the donor's death. Bad things happen and good people die. However, rather than compound their tragedy, a donor's family takes that tragedy and saves many lives with a heart, kidneys, liver, pancreas, and whatever other organs surgeons manage to transplant. It was a decision my donor family made to help others in the midst of their tragedy — and it had nothing to do with me.

I didn't know anything about the donor — not name, age, gender, race, or how they died. Nothing. And I wouldn't know anything for a long time. Recipients cannot be in touch with the donor family until one year after the transplant. Even then, recipients are not allowed to have direct contact with the donor family. All communication must go through the transplant organization instead, at least until two communications had occurred without problems.

Policies are in place because there have been unfortunate cases in the past when the two parties met and one said, "Oh, I didn't want that person's heart." Or the donor's family said, "I didn't want my loved one's heart to go to that type of person." Sadly, there are people like that in the world.

The organ donation organization ensures that all of the correspondence between the two families remains mutually beneficial. Whenever it came time that I could finally write the donor family, I was instructed that I couldn't tell them much of anything about who I was. Likewise, the donor's family wouldn't be able to tell me how their loved one died or share certain facts about him or her. The whole exchange would be censored and edited by the transplant organization.

All I needed to know at the time was that this gift was through someone's amazing generosity.

37

On my second day out of the ICU, Denise brought in my laptop. Our close circle of friends and family (Denise's sister Donna and her daughter Lea; neighbors Sophia, Kathy, and Mary; and Elaine, Lini, and Jeff — friends from work) had set up a website earlier on Sunday called Lotsa Helping Hands. This website became a vital communication link between us and the friends and family members who were praying for us and anxiously awaiting any updates.

From my hospital bed, I read all the postings on the website. It was uplifting to see the outpouring of love from people from every part of my life — family members, coworkers, high school classmates and friends, acquaintances, even former patients — many of whom wrote to say how their own lives were transformed by what happened to me. Other neighbors and friends that I'd quietly helped over the years with their health problems heard about my illness and wrote to say they never even knew I was sick.

This virtual community became a source of immediate and ongoing emotional support, but it also provided a way for people to help us. It was amazing how everyone was willing to do something for our family right away. Believe me, it takes a village to survive something like this. We tend to forget about the power of a community of friends and loved ones, and how healing that can be when you are just trying to survive the day. The beauty of an online web community of volunteers through sites like Lotsa Helping Hands (lotsahelpinghands.com) and also Caring Bridge (caringbridge.org) is how you can organize the efforts of volunteers without using a complicated phone tree or knocking on neighbors' doors to ask for help.

In today's social media saturated world, the process was rather easy. My three friends from work and several neighbors populated it and organized all the meals, visits, and projects that needed to be handled. There was a schedule for the next few months noting meals, garbage pickup days, yard work, who was walking with me when I got out of the hospital — all the things we needed to keep our home running. People began bringing meals to our house every night. We had so much food that we didn't know what to do with all of it. Others volunteered to cut the lawn, shuttle Celeste to events, or do household chores.

Denise's cousin Vicki had driven up from Florida to take care of Celeste, our dogs, and the household chores, allowing Denise time to spend with me. She even cleaned — no, sterilized — the house in anticipation of my coming home.

It was a great way to allow lots of people to get involved with my care, especially those who wanted to do something but who probably wouldn't have felt comfortable calling us to find out what we needed.

After privately hiding how bad my situation was for years, Denise and I had to learn to graciously accept help from others. We learned how mutually gratifying it is to let others help. People want to help in times like these, and to deny them that opportunity is to leave them out of the experience. As Denise often shares with people when talking about our story, no one has the stamina, energy, and personal strength to get through a major illness or surgery without a support system.

Denise and I would learn to depend on our family and friends for a lot in the coming months. Taking care of sick oncology patients for so many years, she had become very attuned to the needs of caregivers in these situations. "Go home, get some sleep" is often the best advice anyone can offer a caregiver. Offering to sit with a patient so the caregivers can go home, take a shower, steal a quick nap, or take a brisk walk outside makes all the difference in renewing their spirits. We are so grateful for everyone who played a part in my recovery, including the medical team, family, friends, and neighbors who came together to help us. When you've been given a new chance at life as I had, it's amazing how it can magnify your appreciation for humanity as a whole — even the kindness of strangers.

I will never forget the lady who delivered newspapers to patients' rooms when I was in the hospital. The nurse would announce her arrival on the floor, telling patients to flip on the light outside their door if they wanted to buy a newspaper from her. For some reason one day during my recovery, I decided to flip on my light. The woman came into my room and we began talking. Our small talk quickly moved to spiritual issues, including how her faith had gotten her through some difficult times in life.

"I'm Neil," I finally said, reaching to shake her hand. I noticed she had little gold angels pinned to her shirt and hat.

She introduced herself as the Angel Lady.

Before she left, she offered to pray over me, which I welcomed. Instead of reciting her prayer, she sang a beautiful gospel tune, smiled at me, and then continued on her way. It was a moving encounter — unscripted and unexpected. I interpreted my meeting a woman selling the city newspaper who just happened to be an "angel" as more affirmation of divine intervention.

Over the next few days, Denise and I began looking forward to the Angel Lady's visits, and we often shared a tear while talking about our lives and our faith. Out of the entire cast of characters who took wonderful care of me at the hospital — a great anesthesiologist, a tremendous surgeon and cardiologist, and an outstanding nursing staff who provided excellent care (including my favorite, Faryl) — the Angel Lady was the last person I expected to play a part in my recovery. Who would have thought she was part of the plan? But she was.

There were also several nurses on staff who offered to pray with me during my stay. Some of the ones Denise and I grew closest to would come by my room to check on me, and they even listened to the song Healing Rain on my headphones. I was always very open with them about how I felt this was my personal parting of the Red Sea, and it was an affirmation to those involved that miracles do happen.

• • •

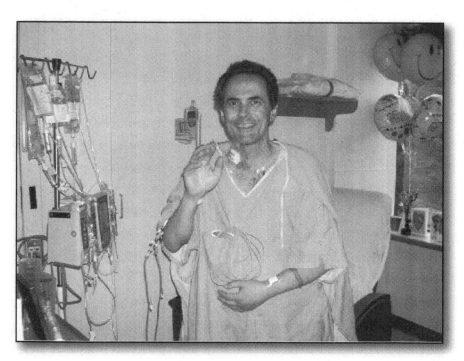

Three days after the transplant. Ready for laps.

I had my first post-transplant test a week after my surgery — a biopsy of the heart to make sure that my body was not rejecting it. The results were beautiful. Zero evidence of rejection. This welcome news bolstered my spirits even more. However, I realized some complications from the surgery were probably inevitable, and true to form, I did not have to wait long before one arrived.

After the surgery, my thighs had swelled several times their normal size. I'm a slim guy with a runner's frame, and my swollen thighs now appeared almost cartoonish. (Like those huge turkey legs that people eat at the fair!) The medical term for this condition is capillary leak syndrome, a common result of being on a bypass machine. During my surgery, they had put me on a heart-lung bypass machine to make sure that blood was circulating throughout my body while they removed my old heart, put in the new one, and waited to see if it would start beating. The longer a patient is on a bypass machine, the greater the risk for accumulating fluid.

I eventually developed swelling all over my body, even in parts where I assumed it was medically impossible to swell to this degree. Talk about painful and embarrasing.

Eventually, the fluid had nowhere else to go, so I started leaking from the holes near my groin where the balloon pump and other catheters had been inserted. Ostomy nurses were called in to creatively position and tape ostomy bags (typically reserved for collecting waste when people have a surgical resection of part of their colon or bladder) to collect fluid from my body. The ostomy nurses had never seen this problem before. I worked with them to tape the bags on both sides of my groin to collect the liquid oozing out of me. I was like a human water balloon; wherever they poked me, I would start leaking fluid.

All this was happening while they were trying to discharge me from the hospital. Complications delayed my discharge for several days but the medical team corrected the situation.

I was finally set to go home!

As a specialist in bone marrow transplantation, I understood the emotional rigors of the transplant procedure, not to mention the potential for serious complications, including death. Surviving a transplant is a delicate dance and a team effort requiring the cooperation of the patient, his or her family and friends, and the entire health care team of nurses, doctors, and other involved professionals. Even though I had a new heart, it was not a straight shot on the road to recovery, as I doubt it ever is for most people. I was fragile. I had no immune system due to the powerful anti-rejection medicines I was on so that my body would not reject my heart, and the medicine also negatively affected my kidneys. As good as I felt overall with my healthy new heart, the reality was that I could become deathly ill at any moment.

I was released from the hospital 10 days after the surgery. Riding home with Denise that afternoon, I noticed how the colors on the drive seemed much more intense. I had driven this same route back and forth to work every day, my thoughts consumed by what I had to do that day. It's almost frightening how sometimes we are oblivious to what's going on around us; we're driving somewhere and before we know it, we've arrived and we don't even remember how we got there.

This time was different; going home seemed like a rebirth.

It was as if I'd never before traveled that winding road, gently weaving its way for 17 miles through farmland and quiet woods. It seemed wider and more welcoming, the green trees incredibly brilliant, and the air — I could almost see the air in the late afternoon haze. I felt like a baby opening its eyes for the first time and marveling at the great, big world.

I had taken for granted the simple things and how beautiful ordinary life can be. Instead of making a mental to-do list or thinking ahead, I found solace just concentrating on my heartbeat, profoundly thankful for and fully aware of being alive in that moment.

We pulled into our driveway and met a group of our neighbors standing outside our house, waving and clapping. They had surprised us by decorating the outside of the house with red and blue streamers to welcome me home. One of our neighbor's daughters is an artist, and she had designed two beautiful paper hearts with angels' wings. I was moved by the symbolism of one tired heart flying off to heaven, and the other heart flying in to take over.

Walking in the front door of my own home made me wonder how many thousands of times I had entered this same door without any thought of gratitude. Seeing our dogs for the first time in weeks was also a special moment. It was such a wonderful homecoming, soothing the hidden, deepest parts of my subconscious that must have believed I might never come home again.

Not that everything was back to normal at home — far from it. Denise had to help me change my ostomy bags (still taped to my groin area) several times a day. My legs were still so heavy with fluid that I could not lift them onto the bed when I needed to go to sleep. The first time I looked in a full-length mirror, I was shocked at my gaunt appearance. I had lost almost all of my muscle mass and my lower legs looked like one of the lost boys who walked across hundreds of miles of wilderness to escape the Sudan.

I was weak, but I made an effort to continue my daily regimen of walking. My father and friends signed up to take me to the mall in the mornings so I could clock my miles. Other friends graciously volunteered to sit with me at home whenever Denise had to go out.

With my weakened immune system, I was in the most vulnerable state I had ever been in in my life. I wore a mask whenever I went out and also when I was at home with my family. I did not want to risk compromising my new heart, and my friends were just as careful to use hand sanitizer religiously and wear a mask whenever they visited.

The swine flu outbreak of 2009 was making national news that summer, and several people had already died from it. Celeste was away at camp when I finally got out of the hospital. We heard that several camps in our area were either quarantining campers or closing altogether because of swine flu. Through Celeste's camp website, we read that there might be kids at her camp with the flu.

Celeste came home a week after I got home. It was a tremendous reunion because I looked more like her father, minus all the tubes and catheters. The next day she developed symptoms of swine flu — including a 103-degree fever. We immediately called the infectious disease specialist associated with the transplant team, and he suggested we get her checked for swine flu immediately (which doctors were not routinely doing, but they made an exception in this case).

Two weeks after I was home from my heart transplant, our daughter was diagnosed with one of the most contagious viral outbreaks in recent history.

On the news, they were warning that this could be a devastating pandemic, and we had a daughter at home with it. I was very concerned for her health, as well as my own.

Celeste received treatment immediately, and Denise and I were treated preventatively. We all held our breath, waiting for the dark cloud to pass over us as we prayed for Celeste to get better and for me to avoid getting sick. Asking an 11-year-old to wear a mask in her own home was not easy, but she did it. We were careful to wash everything, and we sprayed disinfectant incessantly. Thankfully, Celeste improved rather quickly, and Denise and I escaped unscathed.

Although the massive fluid accumulation in my legs continued to resolve over the six weeks since the transplant, I still had a lingering issue with fluid building up between the lining of my lungs and chest wall (referred to as a pleural effusion). I knew when the pleural effusion was increasing because it was harder to breathe when I walked and I felt pressure in my chest if I took deep breaths. I went to the hospital periodically throughout September and October for doctors to carefully insert a needle into my chest to drain off the fluid, a full liter or more at a time.

Once again, it was a procedure I had performed on others many times as a medical resident and fellow, but to experience it firsthand was something very different. Inserting a needle in the chest cavity outside the lungs is a precise maneuver—too far and it could puncture and deflate the lungs, a potentially serious complication. I had several outpatient visits to drain the pleural effusions, but the fluid would inevitably re-accumulate several days later.

During this time, I was also having weekly heart biopsies to look for evidence of organ rejection and to check my heart function. Thankfully, the heart looked great, although the echocardiogram to evaluate heart function showed fluid not only around the lining of the lungs but also around the heart (called a pericardial effusion). I was initially told this was not uncommon after a transplant. However, in October, my doctor ordered a CT scan to further evaluate it since it was not resolving. I was about to get dressed after the scan when someone knocked on the door. It was my doctor.

"We can't let you go home, Neil," he said, as he laid my chart on the counter. "Something is wrong."

38

I was starting to feel that God was playing tricks on me by allowing me to survive a heart transplant, only to have me die of a complication. It would not have been helpful for my caregiver to get equally wrapped up in my self-doubt and emotions.

As an oncology nurse, Denise had been involved in plenty of challenging situations. She has been at the bedsides of cancer patients with no hope for recovery. She knows what a terminal diagnosis looks like. In the moments when I was distraught over setbacks in my recovery, she was the one who figuratively grabbed me by the lapels and told me I was going to be okay.

Denise was a pillar of strength, helping me see the situation in a clear light. It may sound harsh, but the best thing she could lovingly tell me was, "You're going to get over this." She picked her moments. It wasn't as if I walked around every day with my head down, but it's only natural to have doubts when you hear bad news. Self-pity leads to believing the sky is falling, even when it's only a detour.

When I heard my doctor say something was wrong after the CT scan, my knees went weak. He pulled up a chair next to the examination table and explained that the buildup of fluid in my pericardium (the sac protecting my heart) was now compressing my heart. Fluid around your lungs is one thing, but if you have fluid compressing your heart, and it can't fully expand and pump blood the way it is supposed to do, it is a potentially deadly complication if not corrected quickly.

It had only been two months since my transplant, and I was in no shape at that point to undergo another major surgical procedure. But what were my options? I would die without surgery.

They wanted to do what's called a VATS procedure (Video-Assisted Thoracoscopy). A thoracic surgeon inserts a rigid scope inside the chest wall so he or she can see where to place a drainage tube between the ribs and the lungs while the patient is under general anesthesia. This way, they could completely drain all the fluid around my lungs at once. Next, they would deflate one of my lungs and cut a small hole in the pericardial sac surrounding the heart to relieve pressure and allow the fluid to drain out.

Finally, and this is the most important part, they needed to prevent fluid from re-accumulating around the lining of the lungs. This involves irritating the protective lining of the lungs (called the pleura) so that the chest wall and lining becomes so inflamed that it seals off the space, preventing more fluid from accumulating. The lining around the lungs is chock full of nerve endings, and normally the pleura go about their job in the body undisturbed. In this aggressive procedure, the thoracic surgeon rubs these highly sensitive nerve endings with what is essentially a sheet of sandpaper!

I have never experienced the degree of pain associated with having raw nerve endings in my chest cavity raked with sandpaper, and I hope to God I never will again. This is the proverbial, "You never want this to happen to you" procedure. Under general anesthesia, I didn't feel anything . . . when I woke up. Now, that was a different story.

I had the surgery at almost midnight on a Friday evening. Denise was waiting for me in the recovery area and quizzed the surgeon to make sure I was on adequate pain medicine. As a trained specialist in pain management for cancer patients, she knew how painful this procedure would be once I was fully awake. After being reassured that I would be on adequate pain medication, she left for the night.

An hour after the surgery, I awoke to the worst pain of my life. Doctors use a scale of 0-10 to describe a patient's level of pain, with 0 being no pain and 10 being the worst pain you could ever imagine. I told them I was at a 20 on the pain scale. Along with the raw inflammation, try breathing with one deflated lung. The slightest expansion of my chest brought unbearable pain.

I was on a simple PCA (patient controlled analgesia) pump, allowing me to squeeze a button once every 15 minutes to release more pain medicine. However, the medicine had an extremely short half-life in my body, lasting only two or three minutes before the hellish pain would come roaring back. As the anesthesia continued to wear off and the agony set in, I began feverishly pushing the pump button and calling for help.

An intern straight out of medical school was the only physician available at one in the morning (I should have known better than to have major surgery on a Friday at midnight). He was concerned that if he increased the pain medicine I might stop breathing from being overmedicated. While in some cases that's true, my case was just the opposite. If he increased my medication, I would actually be able to breathe much easier. Unfortunately, I could not explain all of this to the still-green graduate from medical school.

By now, I was gripping the rail posts of my bed, wild-eyed and taking rapid, shallow breaths. It felt like a constant stream of alcohol poured onto a fresh wound — only this was happening inside my chest. A circular dialogue between me, the nurses, and the intern went on for hours into the early morning.

At one point after pushing the call button for the umpteenth time trying to let someone know that I was going to stop breathing if the unbearable pain persisted, I heard someone outside my door say, "Don't worry, that's just the guy who has been complaining all night." If I could have gotten out of bed, I am afraid what I might have said or done to that person.

No one came in for what seemed like an hour after that. Finally, the intern came back, after increasing my pain medicines by baby doses, which had no effect, and in the midst of his frustration, said to me, "Well, you are a doctor, what do you want me to give you?"

"Give me enough morphine to treat the pain," I blurted out between short staccato breaths. Instead, he gave me another baby dose, fearful he would cause an overdose.

Finally, in utter desperation after pleading for nearly six hours to get pain relief from the worst pain I had ever experienced or could imagine, I threatened to sue everyone in the hospital unless I saw an attending physician. At six that morning, the thoracic surgeon who had performed the procedure just happened to come by to check on me. He looked at my chart and realized the follow-up instructions listed were not his orders. He immediately put me on the proper dosage of pain medicine and within 30 minutes I was virtually pain free.

• • •

I was able to go home after spending a few more days in the hospital to allow more fluid to drain out of my lungs. It was a short reprieve from the hospital, however, because I was summoned back in early November.

I had already weathered fluid accumulation in my lungs and my heart and swine flu exposure and inflammation in my chest cavity, but now the doctor had called me to tell me I had a rare fungal infection around my heart. Without a proper immune system, a fungal infection can kill a transplant recipient.

If that wasn't frightening enough, my doctor explained there were only three existing cases of this particular type of fungal infection surrounding the heart as a complication of heart transplant in published medical literature. He had no prior experience with it because it is so rarely seen in anyone, much less heart transplant recipients. No one knew quite what to do. I was told I just needed to get to the hospital so they could formulate a plan to save my life.

Being a member of the club gives me a different vantage point when I interact with my doctors. I'm not in awe of them. I like them, I respect them, and I love it when I have a great doctor. However, to me, the greatest doctors are the ones who admit that they don't have all the answers. There is nothing wrong with saying, "I don't know, but I will make certain to research and do whatever it takes to figure it out." That's what I was hoping for in my case.

Why couldn't I get a break?

I actually cried when I told Denise the news. And, I thought again of Job.

There are moments when your faith is severely tested, and this was one of them for me. I can't say that I stood there, eyes closed, saying, God, I know that you are going to take care of me during yet another life-threatening crisis. At that moment, my thoughts were more along the lines of, *Why are you doing this to me?* Why had He brought me through everything that I'd gone through only to die of a fungal infection?

When things are going great, it's very easy to have faith. When you're severely tested, you realize how important having faith is and how fragile it can be.

Ultimately, faith got me through this experience, but I never hide the fact that there were moments that I had major doubts. What I had always thought was a firm foundation of hope was beginning to show cracks. I was still praying a lot, and we alerted people to get back on the prayer circuit for me. I was off the transplant list and they could check that one off, but I needed them to keep tapping the power of prayer.

My faith wavered again.

Someone has to bring you back to earth in those times. Denise did not share in my panic over the fungal infection, at least not outwardly. Instead, she calmly focused on what we needed to do next. I don't know how I would have made it through this entire experience without her. She knew that if I saw her break down it would have been devastating for me. I packed a bag that afternoon, and we made plans to check into the hospital once more.

39

Any heart transplant recipient will tell you there is good news and bad news after the operation. The good news is that you can eat most anything you want. The bad news is there are only so many milkshakes a person can drink in one day! It's physically impossible to consume the daily calories your body needs after a major surgery like a heart transplant. The body goes into overdrive, requiring tremendous amounts of calories in order to resume the process of healing.

Burn victims also go through something similar — it's called a catabolic state, where the body requires a crazy load of calories just to sustain itself. Pre-surgery, I would normally consume 1,500 calories a day in order to maintain my weight. Now, I required about three times that many daily calories because my body was in survival mode.

I have a gluten allergy, so I was eating gluten-free chocolate chip cookies by the handful and decadent gluten-free chocolate cupcakes with a three-inch layer of chocolate icing and a scoop of ice cream on top of that — with nuts. Still, my body was burning calories as fast as I was putting them in.

When I did not get enough calories, my body began breaking down and consuming anything it could derive energy from — I had no fat left, so my muscle mass was fair game. Looking in the mirror was like seeing somebody who looked like me but was only a quarter of the man I used to be. Before I got sick, I weighed about 160 pounds. My weight during this time went down to about 137 pounds. I was physically unprepared to fight a dangerous infection. Nevertheless, I needed to gear up for battle once more.

I went into overdrive researching my rare infection on the Internet. However, Denise and I knew too much for our own good and understood right away that the medical literature was not reassuring. There were no cases about a patient taking a pill and being okay after this type of fungal infection. It was much more complicated and potentially lethal than that. The problem with the infection is that it can cause a hard build-up to develop around the sac surrounding the heart, like the rind in a watermelon, which constricts the heart, compromising its pump function.

Between that phone call from my doctor telling me about the infection and my arrival at the hospital, I had little time to prepare, but at least I no longer felt helpless and defeated. That proved important. My transplant surgeon walked into my room and began describing in vivid detail his plan for treating the infection. In short, he would open up my chest, reach inside with his hand, and scrape out the infected tissue surrounding my heart.

I thought, *If he does what he says he's going to do, I'm going to be dead.* I had that distinct feeling, and everything within me told me the procedure he was describing was not right for me.

I calmly interrupted and said, "No, you're not doing that to me. I don't know what we're going to do, but I'm not having that done."

He looked somewhat shocked. He had already cancelled his plans to fly out that day to see a sick relative in order to take me to the OR.

"You're going to go see your sick relative, or whatever you need to do, but I'm not having that surgery," I said.

I knew deep down that the operation would kill me. Reaming out my pericardial sac like a watermelon rind was the last thing my body could handle. It may have made medical sense, but it was the wrong thing to do for me at that time.

I believe this was my gut instinct rising to the occasion once more. To dismiss it felt almost sacrilegious. For me, listening to my instincts meant the difference between life and death. I think my soul was trying to tap me on the head at the moment to alert me that what I was hearing was not right for me. If I ignored my instinct and told myself it's just a voice in my head, I would not be true to who I am.

The most powerful person in a doctor-patient relationship is not the doctor — it is the patient.

I don't want to convey the message that people should fight tooth and nail with their doctors every time they suggest taking penicillin for a sore throat, for example. I believe in a collaborative effort.

After I rejected the surgeon's plan for invasive surgery, he agreed to leave me alone for the time being, and I sat there staring at the floor and considering my options. The problem was that I didn't have that many to consider. At that moment, my cardiologist came in and said that he had just conferred with someone from the infectious disease group at Duke. To my surprise, I learned that this man just so happened to be the world's expert on the very type of fungal infection surrounding my heart. Three cases in the medical literature, no one knows what to do — and it turns out that the world's expert is a colleague at Duke.

His name? Dr. John Perfect. Another sign from God.

"We have a plan," my cardiologist said. "Dr. Perfect says to take these antifungal medicines." As the world's expert in that particular fungus, Dr. Perfect felt the infection would respond to his prescribed treatment.

I went from being devastated to hearing the sound of harps playing and seeing little angels floating around my bed! Dr. Perfect was here, and now I was back on track again! That's not to say Dr. Perfect's prescription was easy. I went home with a PICC line in my arm and received daily doses of potent antifungal medicine for weeks. It was a tough medicine, similar to chemotherapy for cancer patients. In fact, I even started losing my hair. It knocked the heck out of me. I looked as bad as I felt.

I continued to lose weight, despite my best attempts to cram in calories every day. I feared I would not be able to continue fighting the infection because my body was still craving calories and I could not eat fast enough. Plus, they had dropped my anti-rejection medicine dosage in order to allow my immune system to fight the infection. It was a Catch-22 because the low dose also put me at risk for rejecting the heart.

In order to make sure that my body wasn't rejecting my heart, I had to have regular heart biopsies, weekly at first and then slowly spaced out. A catheter the size of a ballpoint pen was inserted into a vein in my neck and threaded into my heart. With each biopsy, I experienced small episodes of v-tach that brought back flashbacks of my earlier life. It took me right back to a place I had lived far too long. It bothered me to induce the arrhythmia with my new heart. Although deep down I knew I was in good hands at the hospital, I still felt defenseless no longer having the security of an internal shock system if I did get into a life or death situation.

I remember counting the days after the biopsies for a call from the hospital to tell me the results. I never before realized the agony of waiting for the results of a test. When I was the one seeing patients, there were times when I had said, "I'll call you on Friday with your results," and I didn't. I either forgot or I didn't get the results back in time. I assumed patients must realize that everything's okay if I didn't call them. And if I called on Monday, it wasn't going to be the end of the world, right? But when it was my turn and I didn't get that call on the expected day, I was stressed. There were even moments of sheer panic. Oh my God. They told me they were going to call me and they didn't call. Does this mean it's bad news and they want me to enjoy the weekend? Or does this mean that it's good news? Maybe they're just telling all the bad news to other people . . . and I'm on the end of the list because everything's okay?

The mind can be a terrible thing when it runs amuck.

There was a day that I did get the phone call, but it was the kind you don't want to get. Bad news. The worst news possible, actually. After one of my biopsies, they noticed that I had evidence of graft rejection. My body was rejecting my new heart. Since my immune system had been liberated from underneath the blanket of the anti-rejection medicine, to fight the fungal infection, it had unfortunately trained its sights on what it recognized as being foreign, my new heart.

Who among us has not taken for granted the beauty of life?
Squandering precious opportunities to express love, gratitude, or encouragement.
Maybe we need to experience the loss of innocence,
Our impending mortality before we can truly see the light.
All too often our minds are cluttered with thoughts provoking negative emotions.
Fear grips our bodies leading to states of overwhelming anxiety and stress.
Finally, a growth, a murmur, an arrhythmia, a state of "dis-ease."

Each of us walks through the valley of the shadow of death every moment of our lives.
Most are terrified of the unknown.
Few possess the undying faith necessary to liberate themselves from fear and repression.
As my heart races and my life dashes precariously before my eyes,
I make this promise to God:
"Every moment of my life is unique and treasured,
The past is history, the future uncertain, only the present exists.
I strive for inner peace and lovingly accept myself for who I am,
So that I may be a beacon of light to others.
I reject fear and embrace only joy and love.
Striving to be successful is irrelevant,
For I am already successful in my eyes and those of God.
I relish the moment,
For only in the present is there opportunity for personal growth and spiritual awakening.

I choose life always!"

    excerpt from "A Survivor's Pledge"

40

While I was imagining going through another heart transplant, Denise reminded me of a very simple explanation for the evidence of rejection. I was not on adequate anti-rejection medication, so of course my body was going to fight what appeared to be a foreign object beating inside my chest. This was almost to be expected.

Denise could always bring me back to reality when my faith was shaken. There are so many complications I never thought would be associated with a heart transplant. In the moments where I would doubt whether I was ever going to get back to where I wanted to be, my family and friends were there to reassure me it was going to happen.

I knew as a physician and a scientist that things were bound to improve with proper treatment, but as a human being and a patient experiencing all of the oddities that the human body had to offer, I still worried because I didn't know for sure if a certain complication was permanent or temporary. With each obstacle I encountered in my recovery, it was almost like starting over again.

When I received the news that my body appeared to be rejecting my new heart, I tried to remind myself that this was just one more setback in a larger trajectory towards healing. Fortunately, the rejection scare turned out to be just that — a scare. The doctors were able to squash it by putting me on super high doses of steroids for three days. At the time of the infection, my prednisone (steroid) dose had been reduced to a manageable level, only 10 milligrams (mg) of prednisone a day (a very low-dose steroid to prevent rejection). However, suddenly having several hundred milligrams of steroid pumping through my system for three straight days was another matter.

My experience on steroids was nothing like those who say they cleaned the house, painted the garage and redid their landscape. There is such a thing as steroid psychosis if you're on very high doses, and I was already experiencing a sick, uncomfortable energy where I felt fidgety all the time. Steroids can also cause diabetes, which is why I received insulin shots in the hospital immediately after the transplant. While I was on the low-dose steroids, I had to check my blood sugar at home every day like diabetics do. I had never had diabetes in my life, and I did not want to be like some other transplant recipients I knew who ended up having to take insulin for life because they developed diabetes as a complication.

I was relieved when the third day of high-dose steroids ended. However, the human body is not designed to go through this unnatural experience of tampering with steroids. Dropping back down to only 10 mg was like bringing my body to a complete stop in the middle of careening downhill on a steep rollercoaster.

No sooner had I stepped off that steroid rollercoaster ride than I developed severe inflammation in my gums and the entire lining of my mouth. It wasn't a typical complication of transplant surgery, but nothing about the last decade had been typical.

I couldn't chew, and it was painful just to swallow liquids. The lining of my mouth felt shredded. My gums started to bleed and recede.

I had just survived heart transplant surgery, so you would think, "What's an oral issue?" It wasn't the end of the world, but it was pretty debilitating since I couldn't chew and the scale started to read what I weighed in junior high school. I needed calories to help my body heal. It seemed like an impossible task.

I managed to survive the next several weeks on a purée diet. My wife made peanut butter and jelly sandwiches and ground them in a blender because it was the only way I could consume calories. We started shoving whole meals into the blender. Whatever concoction you can imagine, we put it in a blender and I sucked it down with a straw.

After a month, the raging inflammation in my mouth began to resolve as mysteriously as it had appeared. In hindsight, it was most likely one of the perks of the anti-rejection drugs that I will take for life. These medicines also throw what's "typical" out the window because they affect your entire body and not just your immune system.

One of the final mysterious ailments cropped up approximately eight months after the transplant. One evening as I was walking up the stairs to go to bed, I turned off the lights and saw a series of flashing lights in my peripheral vision. Sometimes when people get up from a chair too quickly they may "see stars," then the lights disappear. However, these stars were not going away. I went on to bed, only to wake up the next morning staring at a blurry alarm clock.

I saw a retinal specialist that day who discovered I had an unusual bubble of fluid under the part of the retina that focuses our vision. Fortunately, it was in only one eye, but for months it was like trying to see out of swim goggles with water leaking into one side. After months of taking a regimen of eye drops, without success, and finally receiving a steroid injection in my eye, it began to resolve.

Have I temporarily lapsed into an altered state of being,
Destined to return to blissful reality momentarily?
My perceptions are muted.
Shadowy figures lurk in my periphery,
Grasping awkwardly as a show of support and sympathy.
Surely they do not feel that which is coursing through my veins.
Anger, fear, dread about the uncertainty of the future.

And then,
When all appears lost,
A reaffirmation of the beauty of life arises from deep within my soul.
A flicker of light at first,
Gaining intensity until the darkest recess of the mind is illuminated.
I realize that it is not death that I fear.
Rather, the inability to grasp the totality of life.
I mourn for having taken nature's beauty for granted.
For in nature there is peace and harmony,
And abundant healing energy.

excerpt from "Rejuvenation"

41

After the transplant, I took 12 weeks leave from Duke. However, I still took a few work-related phone calls and checked my emails. In fact, several days after the transplant, I was working on a grant — the nurses thought I was crazy. I slowly allowed myself to get sucked back into the stress of life sooner than necessary. I struggled to put my work in the proper perspective, considering I had just survived a heart transplant only a few months prior. Most heart transplant recipients take 12-18 months, even two years, before they begin to feel completely normal again.

I wanted to feel normal again, but it had been so long since that had been the case that I almost forgot how it felt.

The morning of my first day at the office, I downed my standard handful of prescribed medicine and tried to weather the initial waves of nausea that accompanied taking so many pills. Staring at the work piled on my desk, I found I wasn't able to concentrate like I had before the transplant. I attributed that to still being on fairly high doses of the anti-fungal medication and the overall deconditioning of my body.

I soon discovered I couldn't work a full day. I would hit the wall shortly after lunch when brain fog would roll in and I would become so fatigued that I could barely think about the laboratory and clinical issues that crossed my desk every day. My body would start to tell me, in no uncertain terms, to go home and take a nap. At home, I would try to read some enjoyable books to take my mind off of work and found I couldn't even focus my attention on the page. I would usually sleep, then put some music on and meditate. That's about all I could handle.

In December, about six months after my surgery, my father went into life-threatening heart failure and needed an aortic valve replacement. I was well versed with many of the heart surgeons at Duke by now. It was a huge emotional and physical stress for me to be responsible for trying to save his life because he was rapidly deteriorating. I was barely able to deal with my own condition at that point, let alone orchestrate a surgery date for my father. But my body rallied. When he had his surgery on a snowy evening in January, I was sitting in the same recovery room where my wife and friends had been waiting for news about me. I wanted to do this for my father.

The New Year brought other new changes, and I began to notice incremental steps of improvement in my health. I picked up my exercise routine as I gained more weight and muscle mass. We bought an elliptical machine and I was exercising a lot. I think my wife thought I was a bit crazy because I usually went overboard. If I wasn't on the elliptical, I was walking the mall at 7:00 in the morning with the octogenarians. I was still wearing my mask on my ventures outdoors and you can imagine the shivers it sent down the spines of my fellow elderly mall walkers. Every once in a while, someone would come up to me wanting to know if I had a contagious disease that was going to be the death of all of them. It usually satisfied them to hear that I was actually the one worried about contracting germs.

By the spring of 2010, I was able to stay at work longer, I could think more clearly, and I was beginning to get back into a groove again. I was even enjoying talking about science and the work that I was involved in at the lab. Before my surgery, my mind had always naturally drifted to my work whenever I had down time. I liked the challenge of thinking about all the ways cancer cells cleverly evade the treatments that we use to try to kill them. Then my mental faculties became sharp again. My difficulty focusing had resolved and I found the old me coming to life.

By May of 2010, I had been on an upward climb for some time. I had continued the trend of working probably more than I should have at that stage in my recovery. Since I had been feeling better, I thought it was okay to push it a little. I even felt confident enough to schedule a trip to Chicago for the American Society of Clinical Oncology, a conference attended by tens of thousands of oncologists and cancer researchers from all over the world. Ten months out from a heart transplant, it would be my first trip away from home without my family.

There were days near the start of my trip when I went too far and ended up feeling like I couldn't function anymore. By the time I went to Chicago, I was feeling listless. I wanted to go to certain meetings during the day, but I almost couldn't get out of bed. It was as if my brain and my muscles weren't coordinated. My brain was saying, Let's go walk and my body was saying, Nah, I'm not doing that today. I developed a stiff neck one morning, followed by persistent gastrointestinal (GI) problems. Nothing seemed right, so after I finally made it home from Chicago I called my doctor. I was still on a fair amount of immunosuppressive drugs, and I wanted to see if I'd somehow acquired an infection.

My doctor did not find anything obvious on my physical exam, but my blood test revealed that I had an active CMV (cytomegalovirus) infection — a potentially deadly virus that is particularly dangerous to those who are immune-compromised.

Eighty-five percent of the population has been exposed to CMV whether they realize it or not. If you have a normal immune system, a bad cold may have actually been CMV. Most people who are tested for CMV (all transplant patients are tested) will be positive for a past exposure to the virus. CMV stays with you forever, like the virus responsible for shingles, but a healthy immune system keeps a lid on it and it's usually not a problem.

However, I was part of the small percentage of people who have never had CMV. When they tested me before the transplant, my CMV exposure had been negative. Where did this virus come from? The donor heart, as it turns out. I was negative, but the donor was positive for CMV (like most of the population). Therefore, I was at risk for a CMV infection, particularly since I was on immunosuppressive drugs.

A CMV infection got my doctor's attention because it could affect my lungs, bone marrow, and brain just to name a few sites. It can also cause CMV hepatitis, and it can affect the GI tract, which probably explained why I was having problems. They immediately inserted yet another PICC line and put me on heavy-duty antiviral medications. Just like the antifungal medications had wiped me out months before, these medications took their toll. Between the infection and the anti-viral treatment, I had no energy. I could barely get out of bed, yet I tried to push through and go to work; it was a tough several weeks.

Thankfully, my CMV infection was caught relatively early and responded rather quickly to the medicine.

It was a full year and half after my transplant before I felt almost whole again. I went to the hospital every few months for checkups and heart biopsies, and thankfully everything came back negative. As time went on with no evidence of rejection, they reduced my anti-rejection medicine and eased the burden they had placed on my body.

Doctors also eventually stopped the low-dose steroids. I had been on a proton pump inhibitor (an over-the-counter medication that many people take for acid reflux) to protect my stomach from the effects of the steroids. When I stopped taking the steroids, I assumed I could stop taking the proton pump inhibitor, too. However, this assumption turned into a classic case of a self-treating physician gone wrong; I developed a gastronintestinal bleed the very next day from taking myself off that medicine cold turkey. Proton pump inhibitors block the acid production in the stomach, which is how they protect from acid reflux. Stopping them suddenly is like releasing a dam of acid. This episode (which required a several-day hospitalization) reminded me that you can't take matters into your own hands when it comes to stopping medications just because you think you don't need to take them anymore, even if you are a doctor.

Fortunately, that was the last major problem I experienced for a while. I felt as if I had moved into an even higher gear and onto a smoother course on the road to recovery.

If I learned anything from these experiences it's that the path to recovery is a complicated one and filled with treacherous possibilities at every turn. Sometime in January of 2011, nearly a year and half after the transplant and literally occurring overnight, I suddenly realized that I felt great. It was as if my body had readjusted to all that had happened, and the setbacks were behind me. I was finally there.

It was also past the mandatory one-year waiting period. It was time for me to write a letter to my donor family.

42

Dear Family,

After my heart transplant, I have been anxiously awaiting an opportunity to contact you and let you know how grateful I am for the courageous decision that you made that saved my life. Over the past year, there has not been a single day that you have not been in my thoughts and prayers. I realize that the loss of a loved one is not something that disappears with time. But I have prayed to God that your grief be tempered and that you find peace of mind through an appreciation of the selfless act of kindness that you displayed in the midst of your own loss.

To honor the life of your loved one, you made a decision that saved the lives of complete strangers; that is the greatest gift that one human being can give to another. To say "thank you" for what you did for my family and me seems inadequate. I want you to know what your gift of life has meant to us, and how your concern for the lives of others has impacted not only my life but also many others, both now and in the future.

Your loved one's heart is beating strongly within my chest. I can feel the energy of your loved one with every beat. After the surgery, I made a promise to this beautiful heart . . . which my daughter named "Heavenly Precious" . . . and to God that I would love it and take care of it for the rest of my life. I know what a precious gift this heart is and the fact that the heart is more than a muscle that pumps blood throughout the body. It is where we experience love and loss. I lost a heart that I had lived with since birth, a heart that had experienced much love and sorrow. And I have grieved for the loss of my old precious heart. But that grief was far overshadowed by the sheer joy and love that I have for my new heart. As I have said many times, I have a love affair with this heart.

The past year has seen its ups and plenty of downs. But with each chal-lenge, I have become stronger both physically and spiritually. I coached my daughter's soccer team this spring for the first time in two years. Run-ning on the field without the threat of my defibrillator going off, for the first time in 12 years, was pure freedom. I am exercising like I did before I developed heart disease. I wake up every morning thanking God for you, blessing the soul of your loved one, and being thankful for the love that fills my life.

I am back helping others through my research and through my experience. I can now tell people firsthand to trust in God, have faith. I promise you that your gift of life has transformed the lives of those around me. Your kindness has restored faith to many who had lost faith in God and lost faith in the goodness of humanity. And those people will go out and help others through the lessons they learned by being a part of my experience.

Your act of kindness and love for a complete stranger will change the lives of so many people here and around the globe. I can still hear the words of my parents, "If you help one person, you have changed the world forever." You have changed the world forever many times over. My prayer is that we will meet someday in person. I would like that very much.

May God bless you and bring well-deserved peace to your lives. May the knowledge of what you have done for others help to ease your pain. With eternal gratitude and love,

Neil

43

In my original letter to the donor family, there were hundreds of other things I wanted to write and many things I could not share. I had also included a short chronology of my illness and how I ended up in need of a new heart. I wrote about what I do in the context of assuring them that their loved one would live on through my helping other people. Without revealing too many details that might be edited out, I shared what impact I thought my survival would have on my mission going forward with their loved one's heart. I wrote how ironic it was that I had spent years doing life-saving bone marrow transplants, counting it as the most incredible sacrifice for donors to give their bone marrow. It is the essence of love for someone to give to others like that. True, bone marrow is from a living donor, but it is still the gift of life. Now, I was the one on the receiving end of the gift of life.

I had especially wanted to convey the heart's incredible meaning to my family, so much so that my daughter had bestowed on it a name. After the transplant was over, my family had decided that we were going to call my heart by name, and we thought it would be good for our daughter to come up with some ideas. Celeste came into my hospital room several days after the transplant talking about how it was a heavenly heart and a dear gift that had come to us at just the right time.

"Daddy, I think we should call your heart Heavenly Precious," she announced. From that day forward, that is what we have called the heart.

After writing the donor family in August of 2010, I didn't hear anything in return for many months. I wondered if I would ever get a letter back. According to the Carolina Organ Donation Organization, both parties would have to exchange two amicable communications before I could say my full name, where I lived, or where I worked. We could not share any information that would allow the possibility of tracing our identity.

All I knew was I had an incredibly healthy, vibrant heart — something that the technicians always commented on every time I went for an echocardiogram. It made me feel good to hear their remarks because technicians usually don't say anything about the results. In time, however, even they became curious to know more about the donor.

I found myself often daydreaming about this person — what they were like, what they did for fun, what their family was like. I assumed my donor was a male because I'd had dreams about him after the transplant. In my dreams, I was in a hospital bed and there were several women looking down at me. I assumed they might have been the donor's wife, mother, or sister. In my dream, I was the donor and I was still alive. I wouldn't technically be dead until they removed the heart, so I interpreted what was happening to mean that my loved ones were trying to make a decision about what to do with my organs. I was aware they were mourning, but I couldn't speak to them, which meant I was probably in a coma. I didn't see myself, just the people around me, so even in my dreams I didn't have a face, a gender, or a particular ethnicity. I just assumed I was a man because everyone around me in the dream was a woman.

Apart from wondering what these dreams meant, I began noticing some new aspects of my life that were not there before, and I still don't have a good explanation for them. The first unusual occurrence came almost immediately. For a while after my surgery, I had a strong craving for dark chocolate, which I never liked before. I'm a chocolate chip cookie and cupcake kind of guy. I also began having very spontaneous emotional outbursts. I would start crying listening to certain songs on the radio. There was a specific song by The Fray called *Don't Let Me Go*, and I would always dissolve into tears whenever I heard it. It reminded me of my dreams where the people I loved were trying to make a decision whether to literally let me go. I could be happily driving to work one minute, and I would hear that song and suddenly burst into uncontrollable tears. It was weird, and it happened frequently.

One day when my family was out for the afternoon, I was channel surfing and happened to land on the home and garden channel, HGTV. I realize now that this channel has lots of fans but I had never heard of it until that day. I became fixated on it instantly. For the next few hours, I watched several back-to-back episodes of *House Hunters*. When my wife and I were making dinner later that night, I confessed to her what I'd done that afternoon and told her how much I loved these shows.

I still watch HGTV religiously today. I now love *House Hunters International* and *Love It or List It*, just to name a few favorites. I will actually give up a Duke vs. UNC basketball game to watch HGTV. Before the transplant, those were fighting words. Now, even though my family thinks it's bizarre, it's become so engrained in my routine that I don't even think about it.

These were some of the most noticeable, out-of-the-blue types of things that happened post-transplant that I just couldn't explain. They made me so curious about what I might discover about what this new heart had or had not experienced so far in life. The more time that passed since my transplant with no word from the donor family, the more aware I became of things that were going on that I couldn't explain. As a scientist used to logical explanations, this puzzled and intrigued me.

However, I did have one explanation for these odd events. I'm a firm believer in cellular memory, meaning the things that happen to us are retained within the cells in our body. I wasn't there at past events and scenarios when the donor's original emotions were sucked into my new heart. But I believe those emotions are real and they are still there.

I believe the human heart senses the full range of emotions we express throughout all our experiences, and these emotional experiences are all retained within our bodies somewhere. I can't tell you the exact protein or gene, but I think our life experiences are there and they're there for the purpose of being relived at some point. Post-Traumatic Stress Disorder (PTSD) is a good example of powerful events that don't just happen to us and fade away. Ask a soldier who has been in combat about having flashbacks of everything that happened in battle, good and bad. You have probably had an experience yourself where you see something — even smell a certain scent or hear a certain sound — and you're reminded in a very visceral way of a memory you haven't thought of in years. That trigger immediately brings you back to an event. That's cellular memory.

People tend to think that this reaction takes place in the brain. Maybe it takes place in the heart first and the brain responds afterwards. In fact, scientists have conducted research to study the electrical activity of the brain and heart simultaneously. When they flashed good and bad emotionally charged images in front of subjects and recorded the results, they learned some startling information. The heart's electrical activity actually reacted milliseconds earlier than the brain.

Do these studies prove that the heart is really what senses emotion before the brain does? I don't know for certain, but for those who believe the heart is the seat of the soul, it does make a strong case. Although I had long held the conviction that this is true, my experience has also convinced me that the heart is more than just an organ pumping blood. When people say that a love song, some especially meaningful words, or certain emotions "come from the heart," what does that really mean? It clearly doesn't mean it came from the muscle inside our chest. We mean it came from a part of our soul and spirit that is intangibly residing in a spiritual sense inside our hearts. No one spontaneously professes their love for another person and says, "Well, that came from my brain." Thoughts come from our brain. But when we talk about love, it's straight from the heart. There is no Valentine's Day card that says, "I love you with all my brain." We know the heart is special, but it's special for more reasons than its ability to sustain our lives.

This heart had a history that I was not privy to, but I immediately felt bonded with it from the very beginning. It never felt compartmentalized or foreign (other than the first few minutes when I was so caught off guard by its vitality). Soon after my operation, I began a ritual of talking to my heart each night.

I began my routine the first night that I can remember after the transplant, by putting my hand over my chest and silently talking to every cell. I started focusing on sending positive energy to my heart, and we had a nice discussion. I addressed the immune cells and reminded them that we are all on the same side. This heart was not different from the original "me." I also started incorporating visualization by picturing a rowing crew where everyone is rowing at the same pace. I told my body and brain that in order to move forward and to live a healthy life, everything — my heart, my kidneys, my immune system — had to be working together in sync and not fighting. Does it help? If people can talk to their houseplants and see results, why can't the body receive the same benefit? I believe your body listens to the messages you give it, both positive and negative.

This principle was illustrated to me in a vivid way in the tense moments before the doctors at Duke decided that I could have a transplant. My transplant surgeon, who was the very definition of serious, had laid out several realistic horror stories about my options, including being bedridden for weeks with the aortic balloon pump keeping me alive while I waited for a transplant, having to learn to walk again. But I didn't believe any of that would happen. I was convinced there was a plan that had nothing to do with any of these dire possibilities, and I rallied every cell in my body and every fiber of my being around my conviction. I told myself I was going to get a transplant that weekend and fully recover, and I simply would not accept anything else as true.

I think the surgeon actually thought I was a bit crazy because I was smiling as he delivered all this bad news on the Saturday before the transplant. From a medical professional's perspective, it was awfully strange to see somebody so critically ill seemingly being so carefree. In fact, my friends and I were joking around when the surgeon came back later to see what I decided to do. He just stood there in the doorway, shocked to see a guy with an aortic balloon pump laughing in his hospital bed. However, that memory magnifies the faith and confidence that I had consciously impressed so deep within my soul that everything was going to work out.

Likewise, I still wonder what memories and life experiences are deeply impressed in the cells that comprise this new heart of mine, although I've always been more curious than worried. What hidden emotions may come out someday and leave me with no clue as to what they mean? I believe one has already expressed itself with my obsession with HGTV. Really, why am I elated over a person buying a home in Antigua? I spend the majority of my time studying cancer cells; what do I care? Why is it still possible for a specific song to create instant emotional upheaval in my life?

Six long months passed without a word after I wrote the donor family. Then one day in February 2011, I went to the mailbox and saw an envelope from the Carolina Organ Donation Organization.

I wasn't entirely sure if it was going to contain good news or bad. There was a real possibility that the donor family had decided for whatever reason that they didn't want to write back. To my relief, there was a letter inside from the donor family. It was actually written by the spouse of the donor, her husband.

My donor was a woman.

I sat down in my living room chair and read his letter slowly. It opened:

Dear Heart Recipient,

Thank you very much for sending us such a personal and heartfelt letter. I don't know how to express how deeply it touched us all. It has taken us to a comforting place beyond closure. It helps so much to know that God in his infinite wisdom made sure that our loved one's "gift of life" was bestowed upon someone who has dedicated his past, and now his future, to saving lives. After reading your letter we realized, more than ever, how much God is in control.

The woman who gave her heart to you in death, stole my heart in life.

The letter went on to explain how the family felt that God had a purpose for their loved one who was now in heaven, and that His purpose was to save her soul, and my life, at the same time.

However, it's what he wrote at the end of the letter that was surprising. He commented how much it meant to his entire family to know that we had

named her heart Heavenly Precious. Precious was his wife's nickname —
something he had called her throughout their marriage. When he read how
my daughter had chosen the name, he immediately sensed that was his wife
coming through to tell him she was okay. He concluded the letter by saying
it comforted him to know that Precious' Heavenly Precious was still beating,
now inside my chest.

In a life dedicated to alleviating the suffering of others,
I had neglected my own.
Miscarriage and misfortune
Seemed to characterize my lot.
Dreams so close to realization,
Continually shattered.
I searched for meaning,
But found only emptiness.

Finally,
I opened my heart once again to the Light.
For my soul yearned to experience love,
Rather than unwittingly partake in sorrow.
Where once I had seen only demons,
Now Celestial angels heralded my reawakening.
No longer would I succumb to fear.
I choose to live each moment without regrets of the past,
Or, concerns for the future.
I will live my life with eyes wide open,
So as not to neglect the miracles that abound.
Never again will my heart be closed to love.
This is the promise that I make to my soul.

excerpt from "Open Your Eyes to Beauty"

44

It's an amazing privilege to experience life in ways that most people won't because I've had two hearts. Prior to my transplant, I worried to some degree that I might lose some of the person I was before my surgery. Among the number of new aspects of my life post-transplant, I have to note one significant loss I experienced. It's a funny thing, but I can't write poetry anymore. I used to be driven, even compelled, to write down my feelings and thoughts in poems. There were many times over the years when I simply had to get to a computer or a piece of paper because there was something I had to write; it would flow out of me. I didn't have to think about it or struggle with the words. It was all just there.

That changed after the transplant, and it was a surprise to me because I thought I would have a reservoir of inspiration post-surgery. From a poet's standpoint, I had imagined that writing was going to be cathartic. So far, nothing has emerged from the mysterious place within where my poems used to bubble up spontaneously. I've lost my sense of the beautiful experience it once was to sit down, write, and read my poetry. I've tried to sit down and compose something, but it's gone. My poems always came from the heart before, but I fear maybe that's why I've changed. I don't have that heart anymore. As my old heart, and the treasure chest of emotional experiences it contained, was carried away, so went the source for my poetry.

I don't minimize what has happened to me after the transplant, but they're clearly not the same experiences. Most of my poems had one thing in common because they chronicled the sad experiences of a certain period of time in my life. Describing what it was like to live through emotional despair, heartbreak, and two miscarriages came from the heart and, more specifically, from that heart. Now that I have a new heart, it makes sense that the raw, emotional energy that fueled my poetry craze seems to have disappeared. My old heart found its only solace in expressing itself through my poetry. Every message I put out there was about having a broken heart. I had literally become one with my patients' sorrow. I don't regret it. I'd probably do it again, even though it was ultimately better for them than it was for me to have that level of involvement. It wasn't a healthy situation, but it was what I thought they needed and that's what I did despite the pain.

Is it coincidence that I literally ended up with a broken heart, with an infection that had the rare propensity to affect the heart? Ordinarily, Lyme disease should not progress to the point of requiring a transplant. I'm convinced, however, that it's all part of the message of why this happened. I don't believe it was random or that I happened to have an unusual case of Lyme disease that preferentially affected my heart to the exclusion of the rest of my body. It was a message to me, and now to others, that it's possible to give up too much of our hearts.

Thank God this new heart doesn't seem to have come pre-wired with any of the same gut-wrenching experiences I went through to draw on for poetry. It will take time for me to learn the nuances of how this new heart wants to express itself. One thing I do know is that it wants me to lighten up and watch more *House Hunters International*! This heart wants to move somewhere across the pond, obviously. But beyond that, it also seems averse to heartbreak. And I pray it can stay that way as long as possible. It's as if it's giving me a big dose of writer's block as a way of saying, "Please, don't focus on heartache. You have a complete, intact, well-functioning heart — don't even mention that word in my presence."

When you survive a near death experience (in my case, make that plural) you tend to put a lot of pressure on yourself to understand why you were given more time. I spent a lot of time thinking about that question in the days immediately following my transplant when I kept asking myself, Why am I here? My other heart was part of a great work through my cancer research, and it preserved my life far longer than anyone thought possible. This new heart also saved my life, but what was my new heart's great work? I didn't know then and I still don't know to a large degree.

Life-altering events like mine make you think about your greater purpose in life, and sometimes the answers don't come to you right away. Am I supposed to solve the Middle East crisis and bring peace to the world? Is that what I'm supposed to be doing? Am I supposed to be clearing minefields from Cambodia? I don't know. I have this new heart and this new chance at life. Is it wrong if I just want to take a nap today? The self-imposed guilt can be intense. I survived, while others on the transplant lists did not; my donor did not. Don't I owe something to the world? All of these thoughts go through my mind.

A friend of mine once told me to beware bearing the weight of the world on my shoulders just because I lived when I could have easily died. "This is a gift to you, with no strings attached," he assured me. "If God meant for this to happen, He isn't expecting you to suddenly solve all of the world's crises." If nothing else, this gift was meant for me to be able to enjoy my family and live a good life. I have to abandon this self-imposed burden to figure it all out or else risk living the rest of my life with an unfulfilled destiny. On the other hand, if I don't take advantage of this gift, then I am doing a disservice. If I don't examine my life and my priorities in light of the magnitude of what happened to me, I will miss out. To be honest, I don't know that God saved my life so I could continue serving on 15 committees at Duke Medical School, which is a good description of my life at any given moment. Right now, I don't know that I'm doing whatever that special something is. And by that, I don't even mean what this heart was meant to "do," but what it was meant to experience. I think it's already doing what it is supposed to be doing — keeping me alive. But there is something more. Something from the deepest part of my soul is telling me not to be satisfied with the status quo.

That said, I am cognizant of the fact that there are still obvious risks for heart transplant recipients. I'm not fixated on the possibilities of what could happen to me, but there are times when I think about the consequences of being a heart transplant recipient because things can happen over time to donated organs. For example, blood vessel changes within the heart can actually lead to the death of the organ. I used to be an avid reader of a website for organ recipients, donor families, and people on transplant lists. There were great success stories mixed in with the not-so-great stories that ended in tragedy, and I finally decided that I didn't want to be reminded of that.

I'm now able to do everything I want to do physically, but I sometimes wonder if at some point that is all going to end. Most people don't think that way, except those currently battling or those who have already survived a medical crisis. However, life can turn on a dime for anyone. No one knows what the next moment will bring. In some ways, my life is as precarious now as it was before the transplant. So is yours. That's the way life is for everybody. Although I don't know the full extent of why God did this for me, I end every day feeling grateful for this blessing.

Not a day goes by that I'm not thankful for the sacrifice one woman and her family made on my behalf.

45

What is daily life like for a transplant recipient five years out? The new normal for me is sort of an extension of the old normal. I've taken medicines for such a long time that it's no big deal. They are just different medicines and different schedules, but I know I need to take them to live.

My life is divided into little AM/PM pillboxes. After returning home after my surgery, the boxes functioned more like a calendar. Every time I had to refill them, I was aware that another week had passed. In the first year of my transplant, I could monitor my progress by the number of pills that filled those little boxes. After taking 25 to 30 pills a day at first, I started to see more space in the bottom of the container as time went by and I no longer had to take so many medicines. Those were the little victories. That added up over time.

In the beginning, I felt as if I consumed more pills than calories — morning, noon, and night. In the years since my surgery, I could probably count on two fingers the times I've accidentally missed a dose. I am diligent about my medicines. They are my lifeline and they're all part of the gift. I thank God for those pills.

Today I take eight prescription medications, in addition to a litany of vitamins and supplements at lunch and dinner. For most of the 16 years before my transplant, I had been cognizant of what I ate. No added salt, no red meat, not a lot of desserts. I don't eat tofu at every meal now that I am a heart transplant recipient, but eating healthy after the transplant wasn't a huge transition. I still detest salt. If I go to a place that puts too much salt in the food, it just tastes horrific. I still don't eat junk food or red meat, opting in-

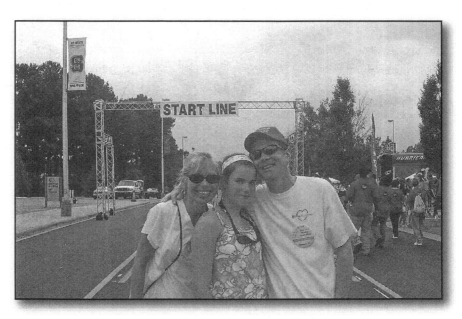

*At the American Heart Association's Heart Walk with Denise
and Celeste one year after my transplant*

stead for fish with vegetables and fruits.

I'm one of those who have bought into the idea that caloric restriction may extend my life. There is scientific evidence in animal models that reducing calorie intake can actually extend the life of animals. Some would say that I'm probably on the far extreme of not eating enough calories. I am also still zealous, probably obsessed, with exercise. There are studies showing that organ recipients who become sedentary have much worse organ function than those who exercise. I exercise six days a week and often run six miles a few times a week. My goal is to keep my heart in shape, along with every other cell of my body.

The one discipline I've gotten away from and long to build back into my life is meditation. You can't run away from stress, no matter how far you jog. You can sweat off three pounds, but if your mind is fixated on stressful things the whole time, your stress will remain. Part of the challenge with incorporating meditation into my daily routine may be that I just don't feel the urgency now that the crisis has passed.

We know we should live life to its fullest, but it's funny how we tend to forget. After any defining moment, we have a way of unfortunately slipping back into the bad habits that we swore we would never fall prey to again. I wish I could say that I'm in a Zen state all the time and that I don't get anxious over the things that I told myself I wouldn't worry about when I was sitting in a hospital bed with a new heart. I promised myself then that I wouldn't worry about a slide presentation and wouldn't stay so late at the lab. But life sucks us back into the mortgage, the job, our children, our spouse, our parents — whatever it is that demands attention on a given day. All those things comprise the moment-to-moment, day-to-day reality of where we all live. Even if you've been through a medical emergency, a severe depression, or even just a case of the flu, when physically you think you are at a point where you can handle it again, then life rushes back at you.

I don't live every moment like I probably should. I wish I could say I did, but that's not reality. I can only try to live mindfully, appreciate what I have today, and not worry about what may or may not happen tomorrow.

On some days, I go from feeling great and clocking in a good run in my neighborhood to being aware of every pain as a possible symptom of something more serious. If I'm out walking my dogs and sense a sick feeling out of nowhere, I'm emotionally transported right back to the summer of 2009. I sometimes get panicky, wondering if I should hail down cars and tell them to call 911 or simply chalk it up to having stayed up too late the night before. This is especially true if something unusual happens near my biannual checkup.

It's not rational behavior, but my mind and body still go into crisis mode at times. My wife still experiences a sick feeling when she hears sirens from an ambulance or fire truck, particularly those that sound as if they are coming to our neighborhood. I don't view these visceral reactions as having lost faith. They have nothing to do with rational thought (like consciously rejecting God); they're not even signs of doubt. If you or someone you love has been through a life-changing, traumatic event, you can be sure that these are knee-jerk reactions coming from a primal sense of panic.

I accept this as part of the deal with having lived for over a decade not knowing when the fatal arrhythmia might strike, and then being within 72 hours of death, and finally requiring an emergency heart transplant to live. Sometimes horrendous things that have happened to you can manifest in ways over which we have no control. But we can't live like that. Long before I faced a transplant, I had to choose between cowering in fright over what could happen to me, or I could go on and live my life. I chose the latter and have not regretted it. I am facing the same choice now, post-transplant. I can live under the dark cloud of fear, thinking about what could happen and what may never happen, and then look back and think, *What a shame*. I don't want to waste my gift of life by worrying about what I just read on the Internet. I choose to live my life to the fullest, not worrying about how long that might be.

A large part of my emotional recovery has involved the realization that I am not that different from anyone else. Life is unpredictable for all of us. Most people, especially those fortunate enough to enjoy good health, don't even think about the delicate nature of life. It's a foreign concept. We assume that when we go to bed at night we will automatically awaken the next morning, go to school or work, and return home in the evening safe and sound. If we live in fear of dying, in the end, we don't really live. Maybe that's the beauty of the to-do lists and traffic jams because they temporarily divert us from dwelling on our own mortality.

I used to dwell on living with the Sword of Damocles hanging over my head. Now I realize that I was living on borrowed time just like we all do, the only difference being that I was forced into an awareness of my own mortality. No one knows exactly what's going on in his or her body at any given moment. Maybe an aneurysm is lurking within, ready to rupture. Or a pulmonary embolism is poised to fly off into someone's lung. Or there is a weird conduction tract in someone's heart that's ready to fire off, causing a fatal arrhythmia.

Each time my body was being electrocuted by the defibrillator, it made me realize in that split second that there wasn't anything outside of what was happening right then and there. I never thought about the bills I needed to pay the next week or my to-do list at home or work. I was only praying that I would make it through the ensuing seconds. Either the apparatus inside my body was going to work or it wasn't. There wasn't a tomorrow at that moment.

Now, I try to remember what I have today, right now at this very moment. And it's a lot. I want to learn from every experience and not miss any of it. I embrace that life is fragile and no matter how healthy I think I am, no matter how secure I feel, and no matter how wonderful life seems, all we have is this moment.

The very breath I'm taking, the very heartbeat I have . . . it's all I've got. There may not be another. I give thanks for today and let my fears and angst over what could happen inspire gratitude to God for this moment.

Because it could all be gone in a heartbeat.

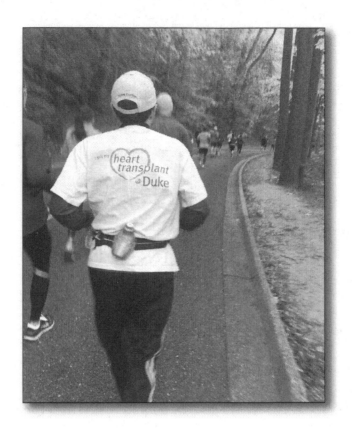

Running a half marathon in DC, 2014

EPILOGUE

The letter I wrote to Celeste about my certain death remains sealed in the possession of her mother. Even five and half years later, the thought of that letter brings a flood of tears.

I wrote a second letter to my donor family shortly after I had received their response to my first letter. That was in early 2011. I have yet to hear back from them. I still pray that God has granted them peace and allowed them to move forward with their lives.

My father and I had a special bond that transcended a mere father and son relationship. He was my idol, a role model in every sense of the word. I continued to take my father to my lab well into his 80s. He used to tell me that kept him alive. He was always thinking about science, as smart and creative as researchers half his age. My father passed away in October 2012 after a short but devastating illness. My parents were in Atlanta with my sister at the time. I was fortunate to have flown down and spent the night with him he died, telling him how much I loved him. I think he knew I was there. I had been with many of my patients at the time of their deaths. Spending that time with my father was a blessing but was also one of the hardest things I have ever done. His death was the first trauma Heavenly Precious has experienced in my body.

My mother lives near my sister in Atlanta. I miss seeing her when she lived seven miles down the road from us for several years.

Celeste is a junior in high school starting to think about colleges. She is an avid horseback rider, enjoying competing in equestrian shows. She plays tennis, much to my delight, since that is a sport that I loved as a teen and young adult. She is the joy of our lives.

Denise is involved in a cancer survivorship program. She's an amazing mother and incredible partner in life. We enjoy our daily walks with our two dogs, and love to travel and think about someday living in Hawaii.

I continue my cancer research at Duke. I am the co-leader of the developmental therapeutics program, trying to bring promising research discoveries from the bench into the clinic. My "part-time job" is helping people who call me with questions and concerns about Lyme disease. I have heard so many horror stories of people falling through the cracks of the medical system, their doctors not believing their stories. It's all too familiar. Eight months ago I decided to get off the elliptical and start running again. I felt the need to run a long-distance race, not a full marathon but a half-marathon (13.1 miles). So, I started running religiously. In November 2014, I completed the DC Half and Half Marathon with a friend who wanted me to feel secure that someone familiar would be there step by step. I can honestly say that finishing the run in DC was more special than running two Boston Marathons, and that should speak volumes to the sense of accomplishment of having run 13.1 miles after nearly dying five years ago.

I've yet to write a poem since the transplant. I have tried, but nothing seems to come out. I have talked to many groups since the transplant about my experience. I have become an adopted favorite son of the city of Tyler, Texas, my home away from home. There's a good friend who holds a breast cancer research meeting in Tyler every year in the early spring. She arranges a community forum the night before the scientific meeting where speakers talk about topics of interest to the community, where I have spoken about my experience and even read excerpts from this book at the last meeting in March 2014. I gave the keynote talk at the annual Komen breast cancer survivors' breakfast in Ft. Worth, Texas this past summer. It was an amazing experience being embraced by these women who are truly inspirational. I am now an honorary member of the breast cancer survivor group. I still see patients and when the opportunity arises and is appropriate, I will tell them about my story. They often look at me in amazement. I tell them that I was where they are, wondering if I could make it through the dark days ahead. If I could make it through all that I went through, they can make it too. Those special interactions help me as much as it helps them.

I still watch *House Hunters International* and still wonder where that drive comes from.

Most importantly, I still talk to my heart at night and give thanks for the gift of life.

ABOUT THE AUTHOR

For Dr. Neil Spector, becoming a physician was a natural fit between science and the ability to transform it into something clinically meaningful. He chose oncology because he considered treating people with cancer an opportunity to be a physician as well as a family practitioner, a spiritual advisor, a mentor, and a teacher. His desire to understand his patients on a personal level led him to view cancer as the great equalizer. It strips patients down to their very core — everyone faces the frightening prospect of confronting their mortality.

As an oncologist and heart transplant recipient, Neil knows something about facing one's own mortality. Neil trained at the best academic institutions and had a once in a lifetime experience while directing the translational research program at GlaxoSmithKline, overseeing the development of two drugs that were approved by the FDA, one for the treatment of pediatric acute lymphoblastic leukemia and another for HER2 overexpressing breast cancers. During the years he spent at GSK and then at Duke, very few people other than Denise and his cardiologist knew how fragile Neil's health situation was prior to his transplant. Rather than giving in to depression, Neil decided to live every day to its fullest, continuing to work for the next eight years in a highly active lab focusing on targeted cancer therapies. His work has been recognized in many scientific and clinical journals as an example of how targeted cancer agents should be developed in the era of personalized medicine.

In September 2006, Neil returned to fulltime academia, accepting a position at Duke University School of Medicine where he serves today, directing their effort to make basic science applicable in the care of cancer patients. Inspired by his own journey, his work bridges the gap between laboratory scientists in Duke's basic science departments with physicians in the clinics so that patients can benefit from novel therapies. After 16 years of declining health, Neil eventually received a heart transplant on July 19, 2009, at 53 years of age. Several months later, he was back at work and coaching his daughter Celeste's soccer team. Neil currently serves as a Sandra P. Coates Associate Professor for the Departments of Medicine and Pharmacology/Cancer Biology at Duke University School of Medicine. He is also the Associate Director, Clinical Research, Breast Cancer Program and Co-Director of the Developmental Therapeutics Program at Duke Cancer Institute.

Neil is more than a patient advocate — having been a critically ill patient himself. After waiting years to receive an official diagnosis of a disease he suspected from the beginning of his ordeal — and having served as an attending physician for the sickest of the sick — Neil understands patients' concerns more than the average person. In the age of "personalized" medicine, he fears patients will receive less personalized treatment as many doctors will be spending more time on the computer and less time listening to their patients.

Neil is a frequent speaker at various patient advocate organizations to encourage patients to take control of their health. "I don't care who your doctor is, or what diploma is on the wall," Neil often says. "Never give up the power of your gut instincts. Trust me on this one — I have a white coat and stethoscope, and I am humble enough to admit that I don't have all the answers. No one knows your body better than you do." Now many years out from receiving his new heart, Neil's passion for medicine remains, as it has always been, with an unwavering focus on doing what is best for patients.

Neil and Denise currently live in Chapel Hill, North Carolina, with their daughter, Celeste, and their two dogs.

43127953R00157

Made in the USA
Lexington, KY
18 July 2015